# USMLE Step 2 (Quick Notes)
# Chest Diseases

- The most comprehensive and up-to-date high yield review available for the USMLE® Step 2 CK
- Easy-to-follow illustrated quick review for the most critical facts of the USMLE Examination.
- Uses effective learning tools, from key facts and mnemonics to full-color images and illustrations.
- Written by Dr. Tarek Abdelhamid (Dr. Tarek*) who is the first person to successfully integrate effective learning models into the field of Medical Education (See: Dr. Tarek's ground-breaking medical educational model: **The Multidimensional Learning Model** [Tarek's Integrated System for Learning and Memory]).

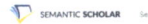

The Multidimensional Learning Model: A Novel Cognitive Psychology-Based Model for Computer Assisted Instruction in Order to Improve Learning in Medical Students

Tarek Abdelhamid · Published 9 December 1999 · Psychology · Medical Education Online

**Copyright © 2023 by Dr. Tarek Abdelhamid M.D.**

All rights reserved. No part of this publication may be reproduced, distributed, or transmitted in any form or by any means, including photocopying, recording, or other electronic or mechanical methods, without the prior written permission of the author.

## Special thanks to Dr. Maha Atout

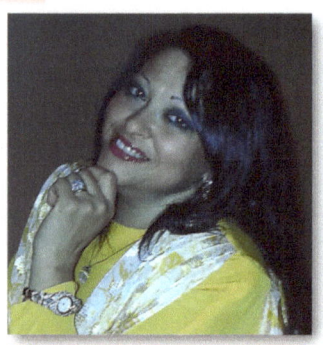

Dr. Maha Atout M.D.

Special thanks to my dear wife Dr. Maha Atout M.D. for her great educational contributions to this book and to all my life.
Dr. Tarek Abdelhamid

## Contents

1. COPD — 7
2. Bronchial Asthma — 24
3. Cystic Fibrosis — 34
4. Lung Cancer — 36
5. Solitary Pulmonary Nodule — 44
6. Mediastinal Masses — 47
7. Dry Pleurisy — 49
8. Pleural Effusion — 51
9. Empyema — 55
10. Pneumothorax — 56
11. Tension Pneumothorax — 59
12. Malignant Mesothelioma — 61
13. Interstital Lung Disease (ILD) — 62
14. Sarcoidosis — 68
15. Pulmonary Langerhans Cell Histiocytosis — 71
16. Wegener Granulomatosis — 72
17. Churg-Strauss Syndrome — 73
18. Antineutrophil Cytoplasmic Antibodies (ANCA) — 74

| | | |
|---|---|---|
| 19. | Cole Worker's Pneumoconiosis | 75 |
| 20. | Asbestosis | 76 |
| 21. | Silicosis | 78 |
| 22. | Berylliosis | 79 |
| 23. | Hypersensitivity Pneumonitis | 80 |
| 24. | Eosinophilic Pneumonia | 82 |
| 25. | Goodpasture Disease | 83 |
| 26. | Pulmonary Alveolar Proteinosis | 84 |
| 27. | Idiopathic Pulmonary Fibro (IPF) | 86 |
| 28. | Cryptogenic Organizing Pneumonitis | 88 |
| 29. | Acute Respiratory Failure | 89 |
| 30. | Acute Respiratory Distress Syndrome (ARDS) | 94 |
| 31. | Mechanical Ventilation | 97 |
| 32. | Pulmonary Hypertension | 98 |
| 33. | Cor Pulmonale | 102 |
| 34. | Pulmonary Embolism (PE) | 104 |
| 35. | Pulmonary Aspiration | 116 |
| 36. | Dyspnea | 119 |
| 37. | Hemoptysis | 121 |

| 38. | Pneumonia | 124 |
| 39. | Pulmonary Tuberculosis | 136 |
| 40. | Sleep Apnea Syndrome | 143 |
| 41. | Lung Abscess | 145 |
| 42. | Bronchiectasis | 149 |

# 1 COPD

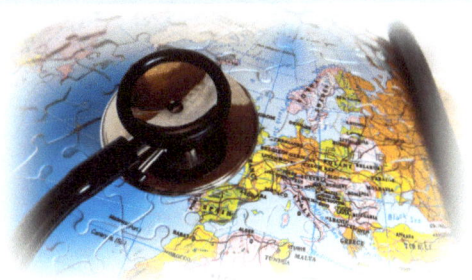

## COPD

**Chronic bronchitis is a clinical diagnosis:** Chronic cough productive of sputum for at least 3 months per year for at least 2 consecutive years.

COPD is the third leading cause of death in the United States.

**Earliest symptom is exertional dyspnea**

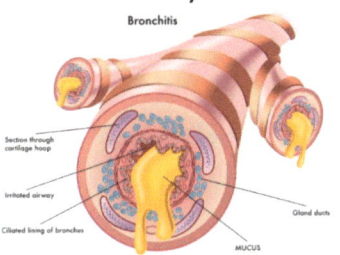

## COPD

**Causes**
**(1) Smoking** (in almost 90% of COPD cases)
**(2)** α1-Antitrypsin deficiency—risk is even worse in combination with smoking
**(3)** Environmental factors (e.g., second-hand smoke)
**(4)** Chronic bronchial asthma

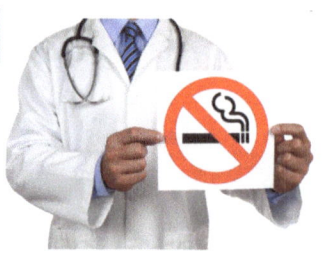

## COPD

Prolonged expiratory time + End-expiratory wheezes on forced expiration

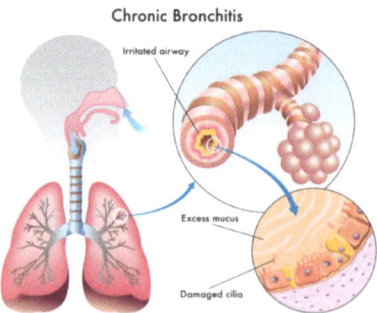

## COPD

**In COPD:**
**The FEV1/FVC ratio is <0.70.**
FEV1 is decreased.
TLC is increased.
Residual volume is increased.

**In COPD:**
**The FEV1/FVC ratio is <0.70.**

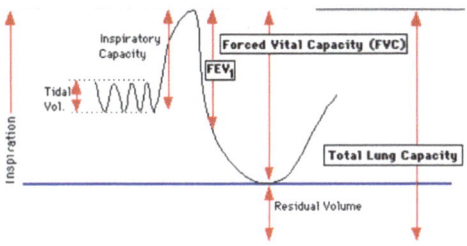

## COPD

**PFT (Spirometry)— is the definitive diagnostic test for COPD.**
Decreased FEV1
**Decreased FEV1/FVC ratio**
GOLD staging of COPD is based on FEV1.
**FEV1** ≥80% is mild disease
**FEV1** 50% to 80% is moderate disease
**FEV1** 30% to 50% is severe disease
**FEV1** <30% is very severe disease.

To diagnose obstructive airway disease - You must have a normal or increased TLC with a decreased FEV1.

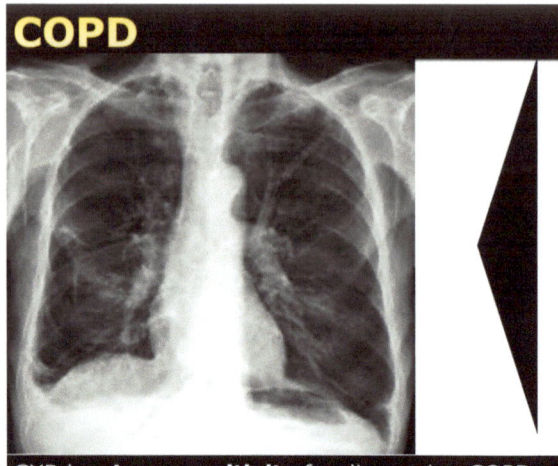

**COPD**

Only severe COPD will show the typical radiological changes.

Useful in an acute exacerbation to rule out pneumonia or pneumothorax.

CXR has **Low sensitivity** for diagnosing COPD

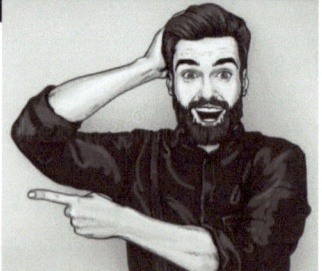

**COPD**

Measure **α1-antitrypsin** levels in patients with a personal or family history of premature emphysema (particularly if ≤45 years old) or emphysema in nonsmokers

## COPD

COPD leads to **Chronic Respiratory Acidosis**.

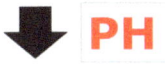 **PH**

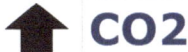 **CO2**

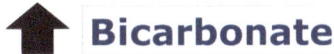 **Bicarbonate**

## COPD

**Smoking cessation is the most important intervention.**
Quitting does not result in complete reversal.
Smoking cessation prolongs the survival rate.
Respiratory symptoms improve within 1 year of quitting.

## COPD

**Treat COPD with** bronchodilators (Anticholinergics ± β2-agonists).

Give steroids and antibiotics for acute exacerbations.

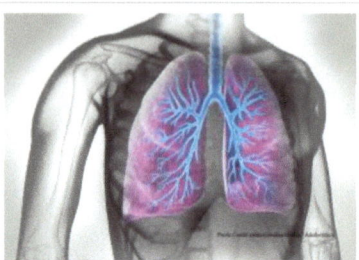

## COPD

Give steroids and antibiotics for acute exacerbations of COPD.

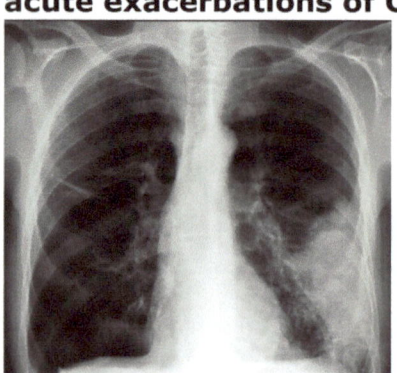

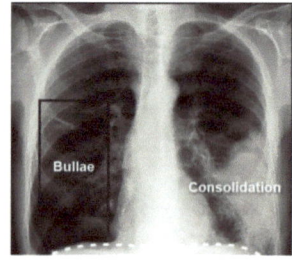

## COPD

**Inhaled anticholinergic drugs** (Ipratropium Bromide):
Slower onset of action than the β-agonists, but last longer.
**Note:** Use long-acting anticholinergics (Tiotropium) for patients with more severe symptoms.

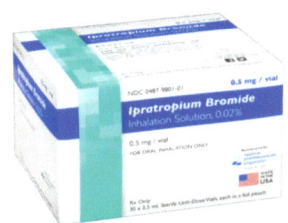

**β-Blockers are generally contraindicated in acute COPD or asthma exacerbations.**

## COPD

**Clinical monitoring of COPD patients involves the following:**
**(1) Serial FEV1 measurements**—this has the highest predictive value
(2) Pulse oximetry
(3) Severity of symptoms: exercise tolerance, cough, sputum, breathlessness

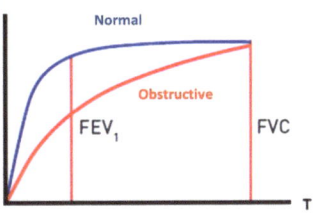

## COPD

**Note:** Smoking cessation and home oxygen therapy are **the only** interventions shown to lower mortality.

## COPD

**Note:** Inhaled β2-agonists (e.g., Albuterol): bronchodilators. Provide symptomatic relief.

Use long-acting agents (e.g., Salmeterol) for patients requiring frequent use.

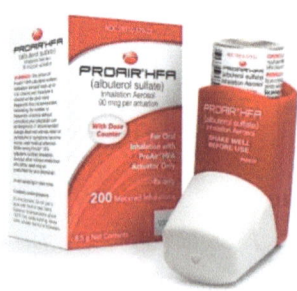

## COPD

**Note:** Combination of β-agonist albuterol with ipratropium bromide. More efficacious than either agent alone in bronchodilation.
Also helps with adherence to therapy (both medications in one inhaler).

## COPD

**Inhaled corticosteroids** (e.g., Budesonide, Fluticasone): are used because of their anti-inflammatory properties.
May minimally slow down the decrease in FEV1 over time (Many studies have failed to show any benefit in pulmonary function).
**Typically used in combination** with long-acting bronchodilators for patients with significant symptoms or repeated exacerbations.

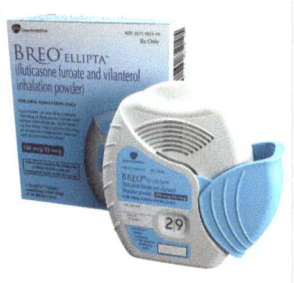

## COPD

**Theophylline (oral)**
- May improve mucociliary clearance and central respiratory drive.
- Narrow therapeutic index, so serum levels must be monitored.
- Only modestly effective and has more side effects than other bronchodilators.
- Occasionally used for patients with refractory COPD.

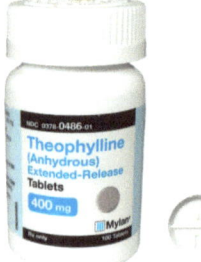

## COPD

**Note:** Systemic glucocorticoids are only used for acute exacerbations and should not be used for long-term treatment - even for patients with severe COPD.

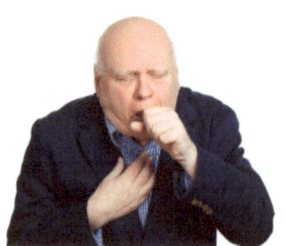

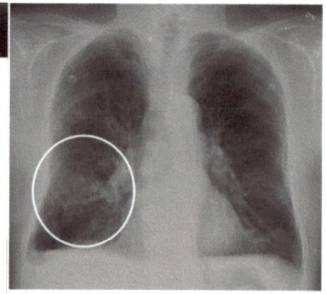

## COPD

**Phosphodiesterase-4 inhibitors** (e.g., Roflumilast).
Promote smooth muscle relaxation and decrease inflammation.
**May reduce risk of frequent exacerbations**

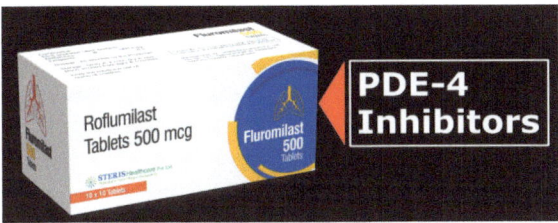

## COPD

**Oxygen therapy**
Shown to improve survival and quality of life in patients with COPD and chronic hypoxemia.

Long-standing hypoxemia may lead to pulmonary HTN and ultimately cor pulmonale.

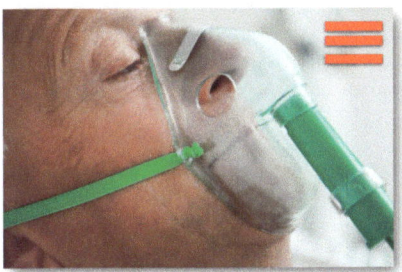

## COPD

**Criteria for continuous or intermittent long-term oxygen therapy in COPD:**
1) PaO2 55 mm Hg OR
2) O2 saturation ≤88% (pulse oximetry)- either at rest or during exercise OR
PaO2 55 to 59 mm Hg plus
3) Polycythemia or evidence of cor pulmonale

**Note** that the above must be consistent findings despite optimal medical therapy

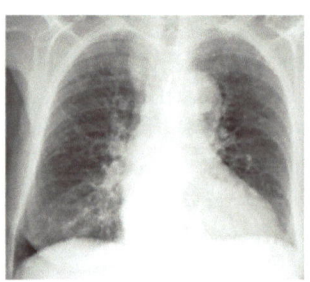

## COPD

**Vaccinations for patients with COPD:**
**Influenza vaccination annually for all patients.**
Vaccination against Streptococcus pneumoniae should be offered to all adult patients with COPD, regardless of age.

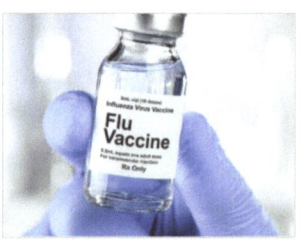

## COPD

**Antibiotics are given for acute exacerbations** — This should be a clinical diagnosis characterized by increased sputum production in volume or change in character or worsening shortness of breath.

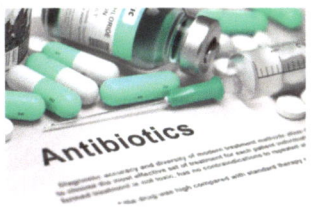

## COPD

**Low risk of exacerbation (1/Year)**
Begin with **a short-acting bronchodilator** (anticholinergic and/or β-agonist) as needed in a metered-dose inhaler (MDI) formulation (with spacer to improve delivery). Add daily long-acting bronchodilator, if more symptomatic. Inhaled glucocorticoids may be used as well. Use the lowest dose possible.

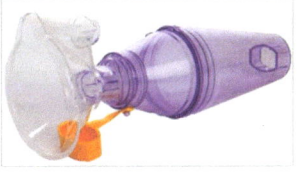

## COPD

**High risk of exacerbation (2 or More/Year)**
# Regular use of **long-acting bronchodilator** (anticholinergic and/or β-agonist).
# Add **inhaled corticosteroid**, if more symptomatic.
# Consider **additional agents** (Roflumilast or theophylline).
# Continuous oxygen therapy (if patient is hypoxemic).
# Pulmonary rehabilitation.

## COPD

**Acute COPD exacerbation:**
**Definition:** Increased dyspnea, sputum production, and/or cough.
**Note:** Acute COPD exacerbation can lead to acute respiratory failure; potentially fatal.

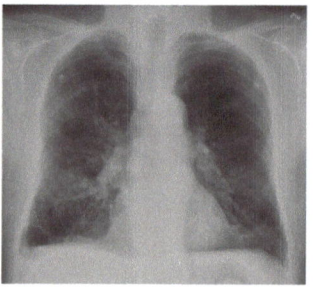

Pulmonary infections (most commonly viruses, followed by bacteria such as S. pneumoniae, Haemophilus influenzae, Mycoplasma pneumoniae, Moraxella catarrhalis) are among the main precipitants of a COPD exacerbation.

## COPD

**Acute COPD exacerbation:**
**(1) Bronchodilators** (β2-agonist) ± anticholinergics are first-line therapy.
**(2) Systemic corticosteroids** are used for patients requiring hospitalization.
**(3) Antibiotics** (azithromycin, doxycycline, or fluoroquinolones): Reserved for those with moderate or severe exacerbations requiring hospitalization.

A short course of oral prednisone is common practice.

**Do not use inhaled corticosteroids in acute exacerbations.**

## COPD

**Acute COPD exacerbation:**
**Supplemental oxygen** is used to keep O2 saturation 88% to 92%. Start with a nasal cannula (a face mask may be needed for some cases).

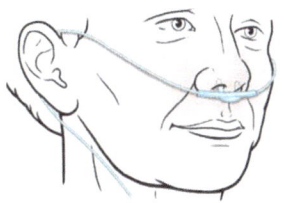

If SaO2 is >92%, the patient is at risk of CO2 retention from loss of hypoxemic respiratory drive.

## COPD

**Acute COPD exacerbation: Intubation and mechanical ventilation** may be required if the above do not stabilize the patient.

**Intubate if:**
1. Increasing Respiratory Rate (RR)
2. Increasing PaCO2
3. Worsening acidosis

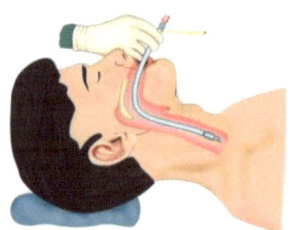

## COPD

**Complications of COPD:**
**Acute exacerbations**:
Most common causes are infection-nonadherence with therapy - or cardiac disease
**Secondary polycythemia** (Hct >55% in men or >47% in women)
**Pulmonary Hypertension** and cor pulmonale

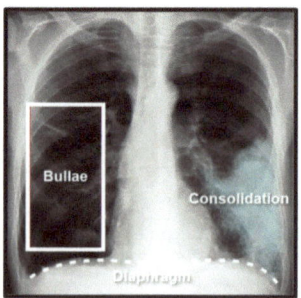

## COPD

**Medical practice Note:**
If a patient presents with COPD exacerbation, the following **steps** are appropriate:
1- CXR
2- β2-Agonist and anticholinergic inhalers
3- Systemic corticosteroids
4- Antibiotics
5- Supplemental oxygen

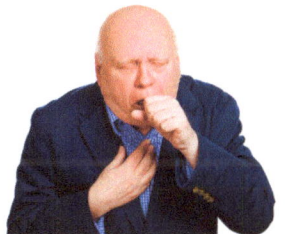

## COPD

**Important note:**
Systemic glucocorticoids are only used for acute exacerbations and **should not** be used for long-term treatment, even for patients with severe COPD.

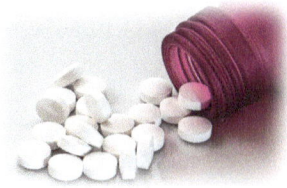

# 2 Bronchial asthma

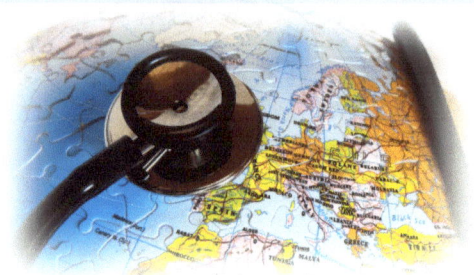

## Bronchial asthma

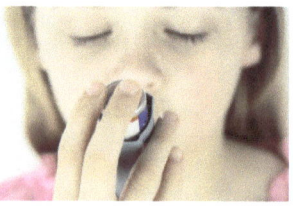

**Reversible airflow obstruction** Characterized by **intermittent** symptoms that include dyspnea, wheezing, chest tightness, and cough.
Usually occur within 30 minutes of **exposure** to triggers.
Symptoms are typically **worse at night.**
**Wheezing** (commonly during expiration) is the most common finding on physical examination

## Bronchial asthma

**Signs of acute severe asthma attacks:**
Tachypnea, diaphoresis, wheezing, speaking in incomplete sentences, and use of accessory muscles of respiration.

**Note:** Paradoxical movement of the abdomen and diaphragm on inspiration is sign of impending respiratory failure.

## Bronchial asthma

**The most common cause of wheezing is asthma.** However, other causes of wheezing include:
**CHF**—due to edema of airways and congestion of bronchial mucosa
**COPD**— (*Irreversible airway obstruction*) associated with inflamed airways may be narrowed (attacks of or bronchospasm may be present: asthmatic bronchitis)
**Lung cancer**—localized Wheeze due to obstruction of airways

Lung X-Ray is usually clear in patients with bronchial asthma (**Unlike** other causes of asthma)

# Bronchial asthma

**Pulmonary function tests** (PFTs) are required for diagnosis. They show an obstructive pattern: decrease in expiratory flow rates, decreased FEV1, and decreased FEV1/FVC ratio (<0.70).

**FEV1/FVC ratio <0.70**
Reversible

**Increase the dose of inhaled steroid, if the peak flow decreases.**

**Peak Expiratory Flow Rate**—useful measure of airflow obstruction. Patients should self-monitor their peak flow:

# Bronchial asthma

**Spirometry before and after bronchodilators can confirm diagnosis** by proving Reversible airway obstruction.

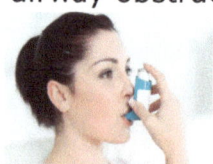

If inhalation of a bronchodilator (β2-agonist) results in an increase in FEV1 or FVC by at least 12%, airflow obstruction is considered reversible.

## Bronchial asthma

**PFTs in asthma:**
- Decreased FEV1, decreased FVC, decreased FEV1/FVC ratio
- Increase in FEV1 >12% with albuterol
- Decrease in FEV1 >20% with methacholine or histamine

## Bronchial asthma

In an acute setting when patient has dyspnea, **Peak Expiratory Flow Rate** measurement is quickest method of diagnosis.

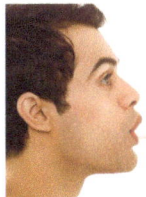
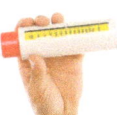

## Bronchial asthma

**$CO_2$ is typically low during asthma** (due to hyperventilation) A Normal $CO_2$ level during an asthmatic attack suggests impending respiratory failure.

**Important note:**
A Normal $CO_2$ level during an asthmatic attack suggests impending respiratory failure.

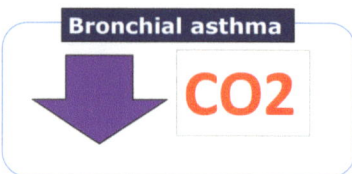

## Bronchial asthma

**CXR:** Only necessary in severe asthma to exclude other conditions (such as Pneumonia, Pneumothorax, Acute pulmonary edema, foreign body).

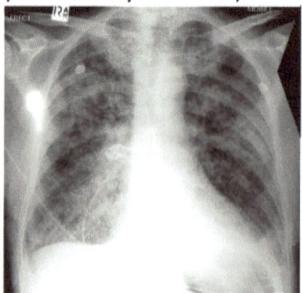

**Acute Pulmonary Edema** (Cardiac asthma)

# Bronchial asthma

**Avoid β-blockers in asthmatics!**

**Inhaled β2-agonists.**
**(1)** Short-acting β2-agonists (Albuterol) are used for **mild acute attacks** (Onset is 2 to 5 minutes - duration is 4 to 6 hours).
**(2)** Long-acting versions (Salmeterol) are often used in combination with inhaled corticosteroids for **severe symptoms**.

# Bronchial asthma

**Inhaled corticosteroids for moderate to severe asthma.**
Preferred over oral steroids due to fewer systemic side effects.
(**Oral steroids** are reserved for severe, persistent asthma.)

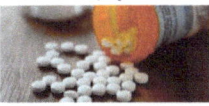
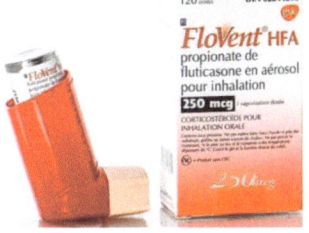

If corticosteroids are used on a regular basis, airway hyperresponsiveness may decrease and the thus frequency of asthma exacerbations decreases.

## Bronchial asthma

**Inhaled corticosteroids for moderate to severe asthma.
Side effects** of inhaled corticosteroids include sore throat oral candidiasis (**Thrush**), and hoarseness.

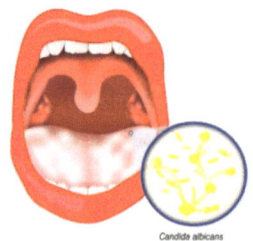

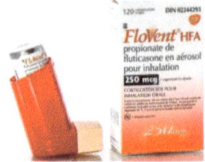

Using a spacer with MDIs and rinsing the mouth after use help minimize these side effects.

## Bronchial asthma

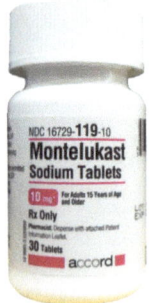

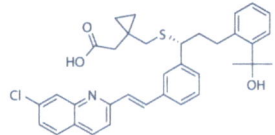

**Montelukast**—
**Leukotriene Receptor Antagonist**
Limited evidence of usefulness but may be beneficial for prophylaxis of mild exercise-induced asthma and for control of moderate persistent disease.

**Montelukast may allow reductions in steroid requirements.**

## Bronchial asthma

**Theophylline**
Can be useful in addition to inhaled corticosteroids for persistent symptoms

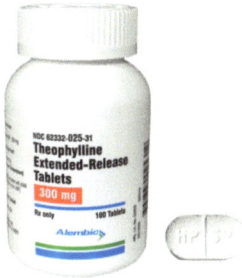

## Bronchial asthma

For acute asthma exacerbation order the following tests:
(1) Peak expiratory flow—Decreased
(2) ABG—Increased A–a gradient
(3) Chest x-ray—rule out pneumonia, pneumothorax

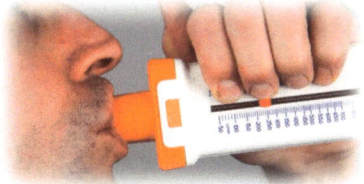

## Bronchial asthma

**Treatment of acute severe asthma exacerbation**
**Hospital admission:**

**(1) Inhaled β2-agonist** (first-line therapy)
**(2) Corticosteroids** (second-line therapy)
**Note:** Corticosteroids are traditionally given intravenously initially but may also be given orally if given in equivalent doses.
**(3) IV magnesium** (Third-line agent)

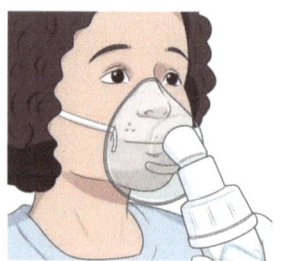

## Bronchial asthma

**Treatment of acute severe asthma exacerbation**
**Hospital admission:**

**(4)** Supplemental oxygen (keep oxygen saturation >90%).
**(5)** Antibiotics (only if suspicion of bacterial pneumonia (as most triggers are viral).
**(6)** Intubation for patients in respiratory failure or impending respiratory failure.

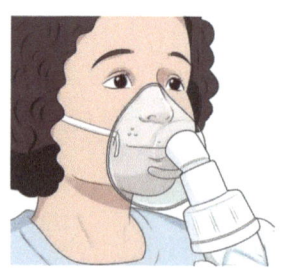

# Bronchial asthma

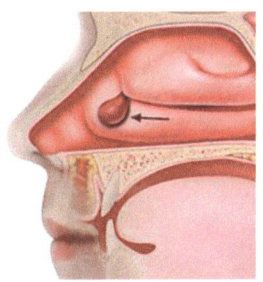

**Aspirin-sensitive asthma** should be considered in patients with asthma and nasal polyps.
Avoid aspirin or any nonsteroidal anti-inflammatory drugs in these patients because they may cause a severe systemic reaction.

# 3. Cystic Fibrosis

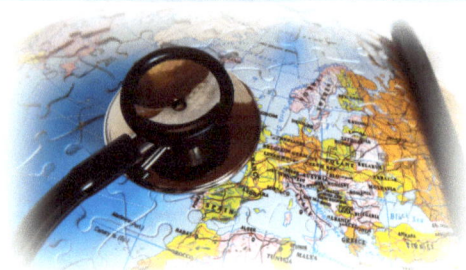

## Cystic Fibrosis

Defect in chloride channel protein causes impaired chloride and water transport, which leads to excessively thick, viscous secretions in the respiratory tract, exocrine pancreas, sweat glands, intestines, and genitourinary tract

Autosomal recessive condition predominantly affecting Caucasians

 **Na Content of sweat**

**Typically results in COPD with chronic lung infections (Pseudomonas!)** *Plus,* **Pancreatic Insufficiency.**

## Cystic Fibrosis

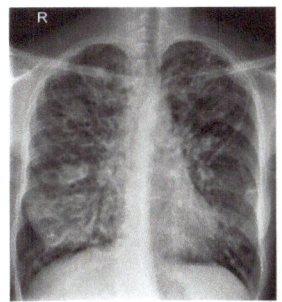

**Treatment** is pancreatic enzyme replacement + Fat-soluble vitamin supplements+ Chest physical therapy + Vaccinations (influenza and pneumococcal) + Treatment of infections with antibiotics + Deoxyribonuclease (DNase)(breaks down the DNA in respiratory mucus that clogs the airways)

# 4 Lung Cancer

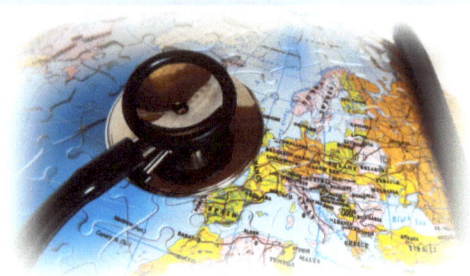

## Lung Cancer

Small cell lung cancer (SCLC)—25% of lung cancers
Non-small cell lung cancer (NSCLC)—75% of lung cancers (e.g. SCC – Adenocarcinoma- Bronchoalveolar carcinoma)

## Lung Cancer

**SSC**

⬆**PTH-RP**

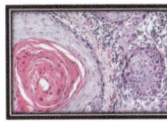

⬆**Ca**

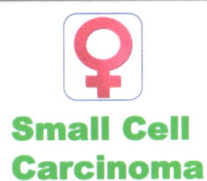

**Small Cell Carcinoma**

⬆**ACTH**

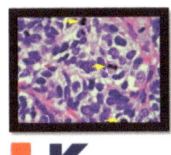

⬇**K**

## Lung Cancer

**Risk factors**
**Cigarette smoking**—accounts for >85% of cases
There is a linear relationship between pack-years of smoking and risk of lung cancer.
Second-hand smoke
Asbestosis
Radon—high levels found in basements

**Asbestosis**
Common in shipbuilding and construction industry, car mechanics, painting
**Smoking + asbestos** in combination synergistically increase the risk of lung cancer

## Lung Cancer

**Lung cancer is a differential diagnosis of any chest symptom and sign.**
These symptoms and signs are generally nonspecific for lung cancer, and by the time they are present, disease is usually widespread.
Constitutional symptoms
e.g. Anorexia, weight loss, weakness
Are usually indicative of advanced disease

In the diagnosis of lung cancer, it is crucial to differentiate between small cell (25%) and non-small cell (75%) types because the treatment approach is completely different.

## Lung Cancer

Facial fullness; facial and arm edema; dilated veins over anterior chest, arms, and face; jugular venous distention (JVD) suggests **SVC Obstruction**.

**Metastatic disease**—most common sites are brain, bone, adrenal glands, and liver

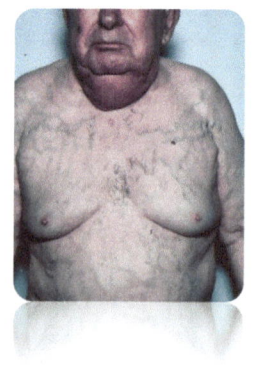

## Lung Cancer

**Pancoast tumor**
An apical lung tumor involving C8 and T1–T2 nerve roots, causing shoulder pain radiating down the arm.
Usually, squamous cell cancers
**Symptoms:** upper extremity weakness and pain due to brachial plexus invasion; associated with

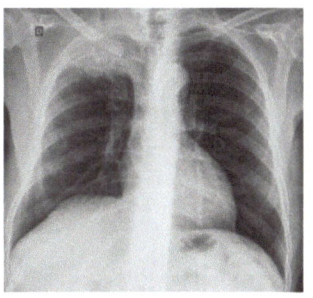

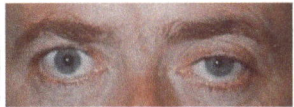 Horner syndrome in 60% of the patients

## Lung Cancer

**Paraneoplastic syndromes**
Syndrome of inappropriate ADH
Cushing syndrome:
Hypercalcemia: commonly due to PTH-like hormone secretion (SCC)
**Hypertrophic pulmonary osteoarthropathy**: Severe long-bone pain may be present and leads to digital clubbing.
Eaton–Lambert syndrome

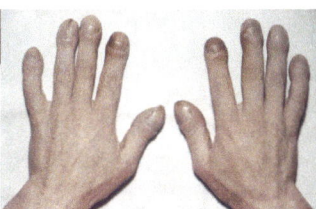

Hypertrophic pulmonary osteoarthropathy

## Lung Cancer

For lung cancer, obtain a CXR, a CT scan, and a tissue biopsy to confirm diagnosis and determine histologic type (SCLC or NSCLC).

## Lung Cancer

**Chest X Ray**
The **most important** radiologic study for diagnosis, but **Not used as a screening test**
Demonstrates abnormal findings in nearly **all** patients with lung cancer
**Note:** Stability of an abnormality over a 2-year period is almost always associated with a benign lesion

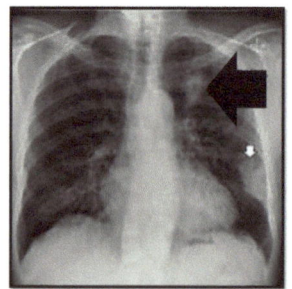

## Lung Cancer

**CT scan of the chest with IV contrast:**
Very useful for staging
Can demonstrate extent of local and distant metastasis
Very accurate in revealing lymphadenopathy in mediastinum
Consider CT of abdomen to screen for metastases to adrenal glands and liver

## Lung Cancer

**Cytologic examination of sputum**
Useful in the diagnosis of **central tumors** (seen in 80% of the cases) but not peripheral lesions

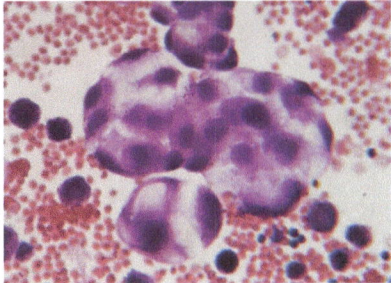

## Lung Cancer

**Whole-body positron emission tomography (PET)**

**PET** provides additional information that primary tumor is malignant (Hot spot)

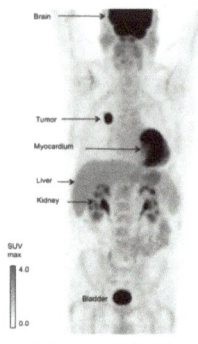
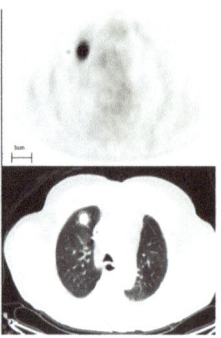

## Lung Cancer

**Needle biopsy** of suspicious pulmonary masses is highly accurate, and is useful for diagnosing peripheral lesions as well

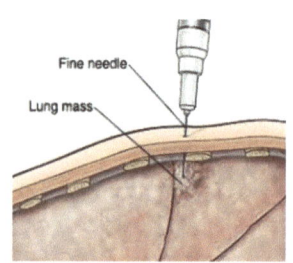

**Needle biopsy is a better biopsy method for peripheral lesions, whereas central, peribronchial lesions should be biopsied using bronchoscopy.**

# Lung Cancer

CXR may show **pleural effusion**, which should be tapped; the fluid should be examined for malignant cells.

Regardless of the findings on CXR or CT scan, **pathologic confirmation** is required for definitive diagnosis of lung cancer.

**Clinical Note:** Most asymptomatic lung masses are benign.

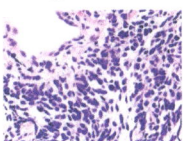

# Lung Cancer

**NSCLC**
**Surgery** is the best option for limited disease.

**SCLC**
**Chemotherapy + Radiation** is used (Surgery has limited role in SCLC because these tumors are usually nonresectable).

# 5 Solitary Pulmonary Nodule

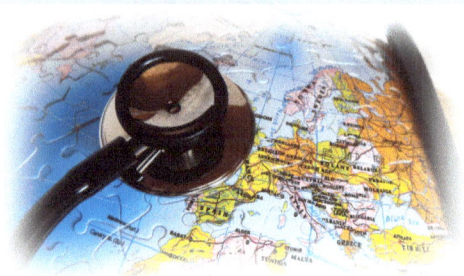

## Solitary Pulmonary Nodule

Differential diagnosis of Solitary Pulmonary Nodule (Infectious granuloma, bronchogenic carcinoma, hamartoma, bronchial adenoma), You **must** investigate the possibility of malignancy because resection can lead to a cure with early detection.

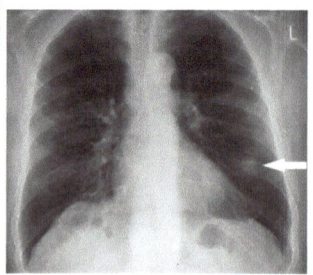

## Solitary Pulmonary Nodule

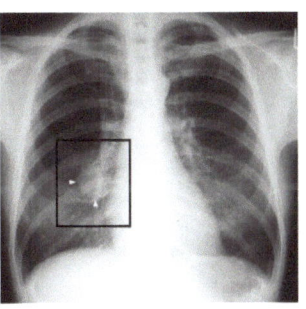

**Age**—the older the patient, the more likely it is malignant—over 50% chance of malignancy if patient age is over 60.
**Smoking**—if history of smoking the mass is more likely to be malignant.
**Size of nodule**—the larger the nodule, the more likely it is malignant. Small is <1 cm, large >2 cm (>50% chance of malignancy).
**Borders**—Malignant nodules have more irregular borders. Benign lesions have smooth/discrete borders.
**Calcification**—Eccentric asymmetric calcification suggests malignancy. Dense, central calcification suggests benign lesion.
**Change in size**—enlarging nodule suggests malignancy.

## Solitary Pulmonary Nodule

**What to do next:**
(1) **Low**-probability nodules: Serial CT scan
(2) **Intermediate**-probability nodule, 1 cm or larger: PET scan. If PET positive, perform lung biopsy
(3) **High**-probability nodule: Biopsy followed by lobectomy, if appropriate.

## Solitary Pulmonary Nodule

**Previous CXR is very helpful in evaluating lung nodules:** Every effort should be made to find a previous CXR for comparison. If the lesion is stable for more than 2 years, it is likely benign.
Malignant lesions grow relatively rapidly (usually evident within months).

**Growth over a period of days** is usually benign (Often infectious/inflammatory)

If the lesion is stable for more than 2 years, it is likely to be benign.

# 6 Mediastinal Masses

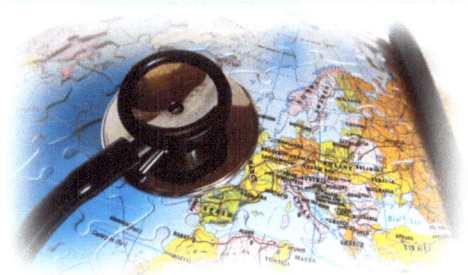

## Mediastinal Masses

Usually discovered incidentally on a CXR performed for another reason
**Chest CT with IV contrast is test of choice**
If CT scan suggests a benign mass and the patient is asymptomatic, observation is appropriate.

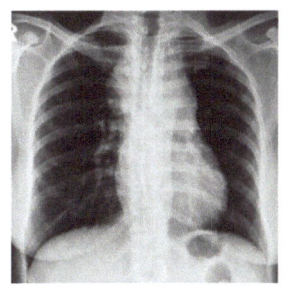

## Mediastinal Masses

In adults, the most common causes of a mediastinal masses are:
**Anterior mediastinum:** Thymomas and lymphomas (both Hodgkin and non-Hodgkin)
**Middle mediastinum:** Lymph node enlargement and vascular masses
**Posterior mediastinum:** Neurogenic tumors and esophageal abnormalities

In children, the most common mediastinal masses are neurogenic tumors and cysts.

## Mediastinal Masses

**Anterior mediastinum**
Aneurysm
Angiomatous tumor
Goiter
Lipoma
Lymphoma
Morgagni hernia
Parathyroid tumor
Pericardial cyst
Teratoma
Thymoma
Thyroid tumor

**Middle mediastinum**
Bronchogenic cyst
Bronchogenic tumor
Lymph node hyperplasia
Lymphoma
Pleuropericardial cyst
Vascular masses

Labels on diagram: Trachea, Esophagus, Aorta, Heart in pericardium, Diaphragm

**Posterior mediastinum**
Aneurysm
Bronchogenic tumor
Enteric cyst
Esophageal diverticula
Esophageal tumor
Neurogenic tumor

**Possible Causes of a Mediastinal Mass:**

# 7 Dry pleurisy

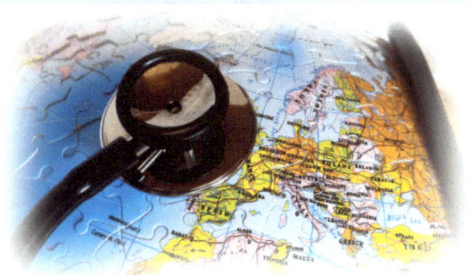

## Dry pleurisy

**Coxsackie Virus**
One of the most common causes of pleurisy- May start as Influenza Like- attack followed by chest pain- May cause aseptic meningitis and orchitic
Associated with: **Chest pain**-Dry cough- Pleural Rub.

**Localized- Stitching- Do not radiate except in basal pleurisy (epigastrium and Left shoulder) - Increase by: Inspiration-Cough- Strain- Decrease by: Holding respiration or Fixing the affected side (Patient prefer to sleep of the affected side)**

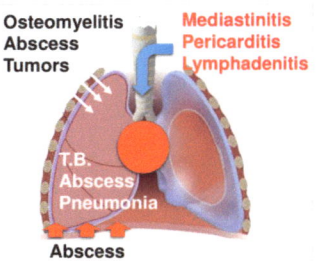

## Dry pleurisy

❶ Analgesics (such as Indomethacin)
❷ Codeine
To suppress the irritative cough if retention of airway secretions is
NOT a likely complication
❸ Nerve block may be needed in some cases to control the pain
*Plus*, treatment of the cause.

**In patients with COPD:** Pleuritic chest pain limits chest expansion and thus may lead to Respiratory failure in such patients.

 **Treatment of pleurisy**

**Causes of pleurisy include:**
Viruses- RA- SLE- Uremia

# 8 Pleural Effusion

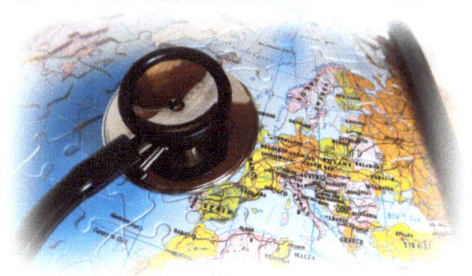

## Pleural Effusion

**Causes of Pleural Effusion:**
**CHF is the most common cause of pleural effusion**
Pneumonia (bacterial)
Malignancies: lung (36%), breast (25%), lymphoma (10%)
Pulmonary embolism (PE)
Viral diseases
Cirrhosis with ascites (also known as hepatic hydrothorax)

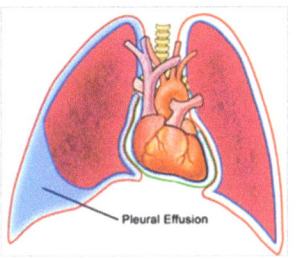

## Pleural Effusion

**DD of Pleural effusion:**
(1) Elevated pleural fluid amylase: esophageal rupture, pancreatitis, malignancy
(2) Milky, opalescent fluid: chylothorax (lymph in the pleural space)
(3) Frankly purulent fluid: empyema (pus in the pleural space)
(4) Bloody effusion: malignancy
(5) Exudative effusions that are primarily lymphocytic: TB
(6) pH <7.2: parapneumonic effusion or empyema

## Pleural Effusion

**Pleural effusion in presence of pneumonia**
Uncomplicated effusions: antibiotics alone are sufficient (in most cases)
Complicated effusions or empyema need Chest tube drainage

**Surgical lysis of adhesions may be required in some cases of empyema**

Intrapleural injection of fibrinolytic agents (streptokinase, urokinase, or tissue plasminogen activator [tPA]); may accelerate the drainage of empyema.

## Pleural Effusion

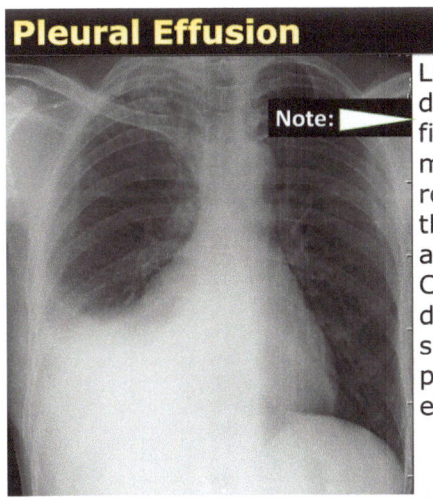

Note: Lateral decubitus films: more reliable than PA and lateral CXRs for detecting small pleural effusions.

**CT chest**—more reliable than CXR for detecting effusions

## Pleural Effusion

**Transudative effusions**
CHF
Cirrhosis
PE
Nephrotic syndrome
Peritoneal dialysis
Hypoalbuminemia
Atelectasis

Straw Yellow
⬇ SG
⬇ Proteins
⬇ Cells:

**Treatment**
Diuretics and Sodium restriction
Therapeutic thoracentesis—only if massive effusion is causing dyspnea

## Pleural Effusion
### Exudative
Bacterial pneumonia, TB
Malignancy, metastatic disease
Viral infection
PE
Collagen vascular diseases

**Treat underlying disease**

Straw Yellow
⬆ SG
⬆ Proteins
⬆ Cells: Lymphocytes

# 9 Empyema

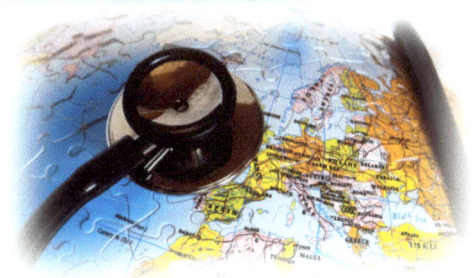

## Empyema

# Most cases occur as a complication of **bacterial pneumonia**, but other foci of infection can also spread to the pleural space (e.g., mediastinitis, abscess).
# CXR and CT scan of the chest are the recommended tests.
# Treat empyema with aggressive drainage of the pleura (via thoracentesis) and antibiotic therapy.

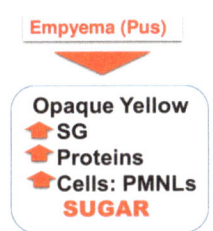

Empyema (Pus)
↓
Opaque Yellow
⬆ SG
⬆ Proteins
⬆ Cells: PMNLs
**SUGAR**

# 10 Pneumothorax

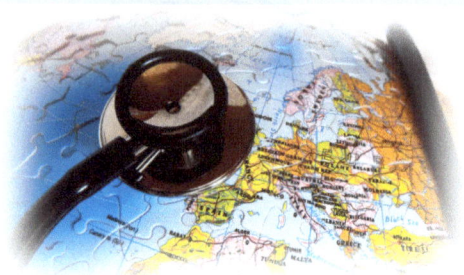

## Pneumothorax

### Secondary (complicated) pneumothorax
Occurs as a complication of **underlying lung disease**, most commonly **COPD**; other underlying conditions include asthma, interstitial lung disease (ILD), neoplasms, CF, and tuberculosis (TB)

Is more life-threatening than spontaneous pneumothorax because of lack of pulmonary reserve in these patients

### Spontaneous pneumothorax
Occurs without any trauma.
More common in tall, lean young men.
No severe respiratory distress in most cases.
Recurrence rate is high.

## Pneumothorax

**Clinical Features**
Ipsilateral chest pain, usually sudden in onset- Dyspnea- Cough
Decreased breath sounds over the affected side
Hyperresonance over the chest
Decreased or absent tactile fremitus on the affected side
Mediastinal shift toward the side of the pneumothorax

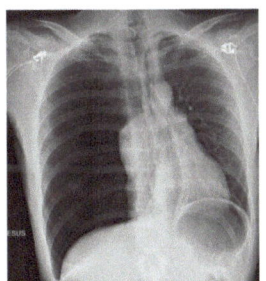

**CXR confirms the diagnosis**

## Pneumothorax

**If pneumothorax is small and patient is asymptomatic:**
**Observation**—should resolve spontaneously in approximately 10 days

## Pneumothorax

**If pneumothorax is larger and/or patient is symptomatic:**
1) Administration of supplemental oxygen, which helps with resorption of pleural air
2) Needle aspiration or chest tube insertion to allow air to be released and lung to re-expand.

## Pneumothorax

**Secondary spontaneous Pneumothorax—**
Treatment is chest tube drainage Plus treatment of the cause.

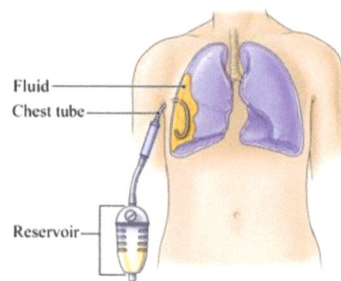

# 11 Tension Pneumothorax

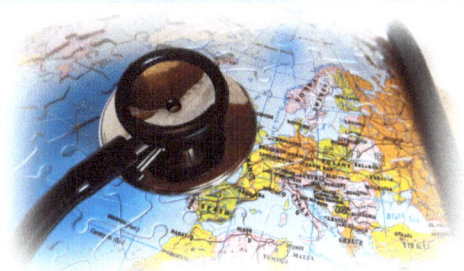

## Tension Pneumothorax

### Must be treated as Medical Emergency

**Clinical Manifestations:**
Severe progressive dyspnea
Hypotension
Distended neck veins
Shift of trachea away from the side of the pneumothorax on CXR
Decreased breath sounds on the affected side
Hyperresonance to percussion on the side of the pneumothorax

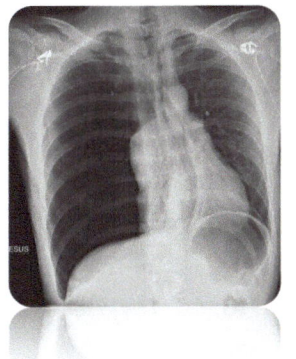

## Tension Pneumothorax

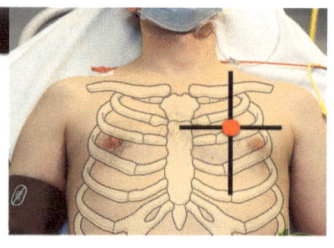

**Note:** Do not wait to obtain CXR if a tension pneumothorax is suspected - **Immediately perform chest decompression** with a large-bore needle (In the second intercostal space in the midclavicular line)- followed immediately by chest tube placement.

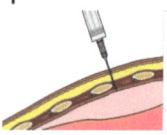

Do not wait to obtain CXR if a tension pneumothorax is suspected.

# 12 Malignant Mesothelioma

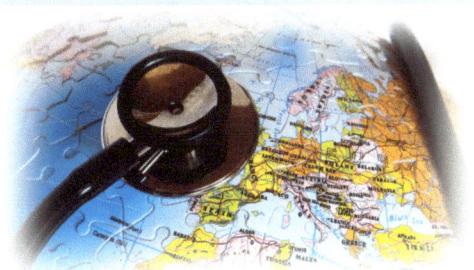

## Malignant Mesothelioma

Most cases are secondary to **asbestos exposure**.
Dyspnea, weight loss, and cough are common findings.
Bloody effusion is common.
Prognosis is dismal (few months' survival).

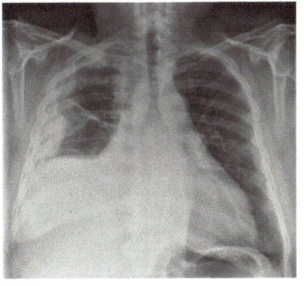

# 13 Interstitial Lung Disease (ILD)

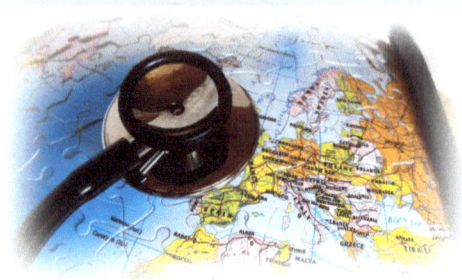

## Interstitial Lung Disease

❶ **If ILD is suspected, ask about the following:**
**Medication history**, because some drugs are known to be toxic to lungs (e.g., chemotherapeutic agents, gold, amiodarone, penicillamine, and nitrofurantoin)

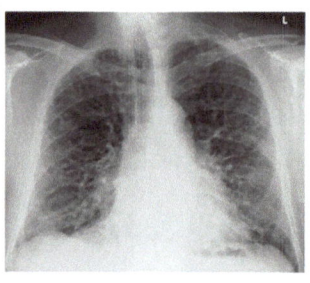

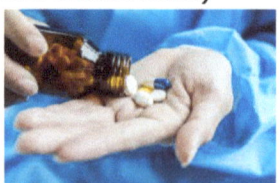

## Interstitial Lung Disease

**❷ If ILD is suspected, ask about the following:**
**Previous jobs**, because occupational exposure is a cause of ILD (asbestos, silicone, beryllium, coal)

## Interstitial Lung Disease

**❸ If ILD is suspected, ask about the following:**
**Past medical history**, as many conditions are associated with ILD (Connective tissue disease, inflammatory bowel disease, allergic rhinitis/asthma)

## Interstitial Lung Disease
**Symptoms**
Dyspnea (at first with exertion; later at rest)
Cough (nonproductive)
Fatigue
Other symptoms may be present secondary to another condition (such as a connective tissue disorder)

## Interstitial Lung Disease
**Signs**
Rales at the bases are common
Digital clubbing is common (especially with idiopathic pulmonary fibrosis)
Signs of pulmonary HTN and cyanosis in advanced disease

## Interstitial Lung Disease
1- CXR
2- High-resolution CT scan
3- PFTs
**A restrictive pattern is noted:** All lung volumes are low. Both FEV1 and FVC are reduced, but the ratio is often preserved.
4- Low diffusing capacity (DLCO).
5- Oxygen desaturation during exercise.

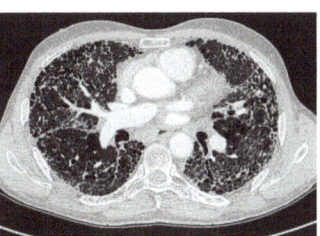

## Interstitial Lung Disease
1- CXR
2- High-resolution CT scan
3- PFTs
A restrictive pattern is noted: All lung volumes are low. Both FEV1 and FVC are reduced, but the ratio is often preserved.
4- Low diffusing capacity (DLCO).
5- Oxygen desaturation during exercise.

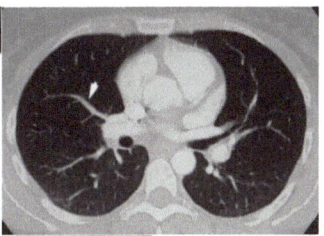

## ILD- Idiopathic IPF

- Dyspnea
- Non-Productive Cough
- Basal late crackles
- Clubbing of fingers
- Pulmonary Hypertension (Late)
- Ground Glass Appearance......
- Honey Comb Appearance [Later]
- Lung biopsy is diagnostic

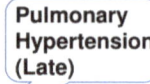
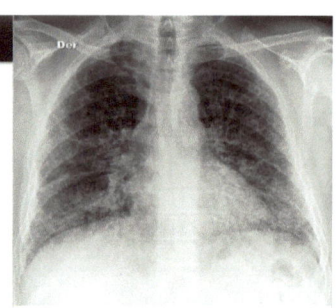

**Treatment include Corticosteroids - Interferon - Cyclosporine**

## ILD- Asbestosis

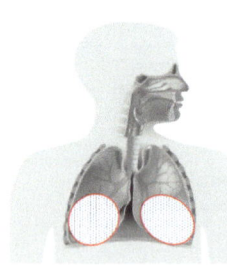
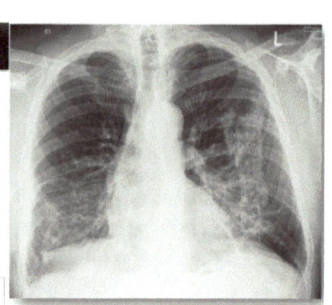

- More in lower lung lobes
- Pleural Plaques (**NOT** premalignant)
- **Mesothelioma**
- Increase Incidence of lung cancer

## ILD- Silicosis

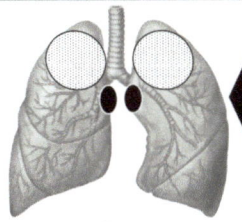 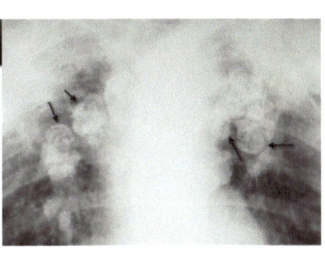

Initial lesion appears as Miliary infiltration of upper lung lobes

**Egg shell Calcification**

**If the patient developed Hemoptysis plus Loss of weight suspect Tuberculosis**

# 14 Sarcoidosis

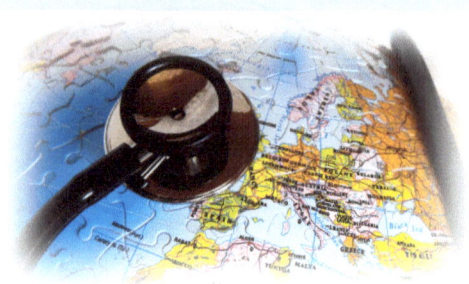

## Sarcoidosis

**Clinical features**
Constitutional symptoms
Malaise, fever, anorexia, weight loss
Erythema nodosum
Anterior uveitis
Conduction disturbances, such as heart block
Arthralgias and arthritis
Cranial nerve VII involvement (Bell palsy)
Peripheral neuropathy

Cardiac disease is the most common cause of death in patients with sarcoidosis.

10% to 20% of patients with sarcoidosis are asymptomatic

## Sarcoidosis

Diagnosis is based on clinical, radiographic, and histologic findings.
**CXR**—Bilateral hilar adenopathy is the hallmark of this disease but is not specific; it is seen in 50% of cases.

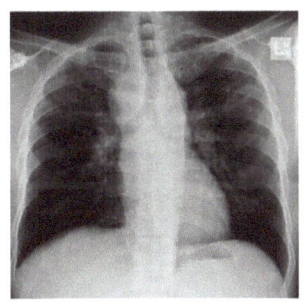

**Skin anergy** with tuberculin skin test—typical finding but not diagnostic

Angiotensin-converting enzyme (**ACE**) is elevated in serum in about 70% of patients. However, it lacks sensitivity and specificity.

## Sarcoidosis

Hypercalciuria and hypercalcemia are common (Due to increase local production of vitamin D by the granuloma).
**Definitive diagnosis requires biopsy.**
You must see noncaseating granulomas- Not diagnostic and must be used in the context of the clinical presentation.

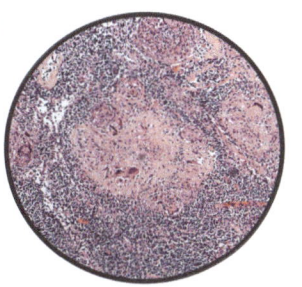

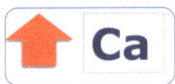

## Sarcoidosis

**Typical presentation of sarcoidosis:**

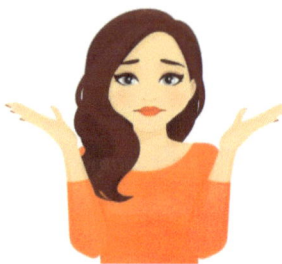
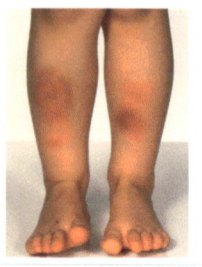
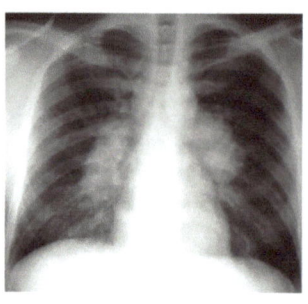

Young patient with constitutional symptoms, respiratory complaints, erythema nodosum, blurred vision, and bilateral hilar adenopathy.

## Sarcoidosis

**Most** cases of sarcoidosis resolve spontaneously in 2 years and do not require treatment.
**Systemic corticosteroids are the treatment of choice.**

Methotrexate can be used in patients with progressive disease refractory to corticosteroids.

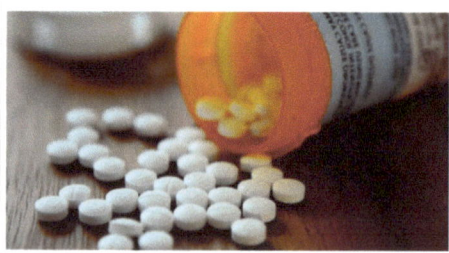

# 15. Pulmonary Langerhans Cell Histiocytosis

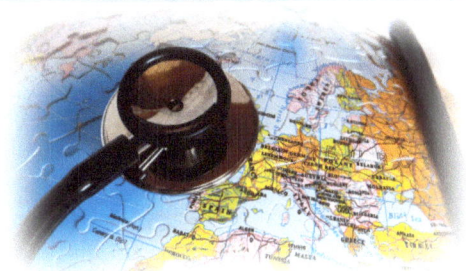

## Pulmonary Langerhans Cell Histiocytosis

Chronic interstitial pneumonia caused by **abnormal proliferation of histiocytes**.

Most patients (90%) are **cigarette smokers.**

Common findings include dyspnea and nonproductive cough.

CXR has a honeycomb appearance, and CT scan shows cystic lesions.

Corticosteroids are sometimes effective.

Other possible manifestations are spontaneous pneumothorax, lytic bone lesions, and diabetes insipidus.

# 16. Wegener Granulomatosis

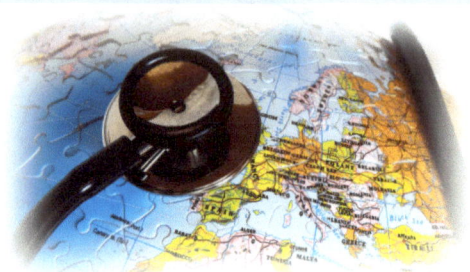

## Wegener Granulomatosis
**Necrotizing granulomatous vasculitis.**
Affects vessels of lungs, kidneys, upper airway, skin, and sometimes other organs.
Manifestations include upper and lower respiratory infections, glomerulonephritis, and pulmonary nodules.
Biopsy is diagnostic.
Positive C-antineutrophil cytoplasmic antibodies

## Granulomatosis With Polyangiitis
Treatment usually includes immunosuppressive agents *Plus* glucocorticoids.

# 17 Churg–Strauss Syndrome

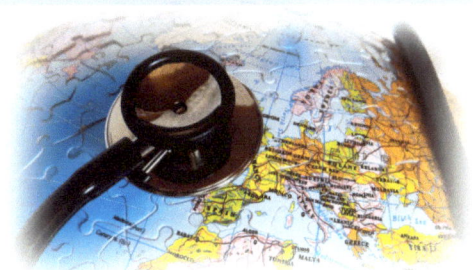

## Churg–Strauss Syndrome

Granulomatous vasculitis is seen in patients with **asthma**. Typically presents with pulmonary infiltrates, rash, and **eosinophilia**. Systemic vasculitis may result in skin, muscle, and nerve lesions. Associated with perinuclear antineutrophil cytoplasmic antibody. Diagnosis is based on clinical findings + Significant eosinophilia. Treatment is systemic glucocorticoids.

Eosinophilic Granulomatosis With Polyangiitis
**Diagnosis is based on clinical findings + Significant eosinophilia.**

# 18 Antineutrophil cytoplasmic antibodies (ANCA)

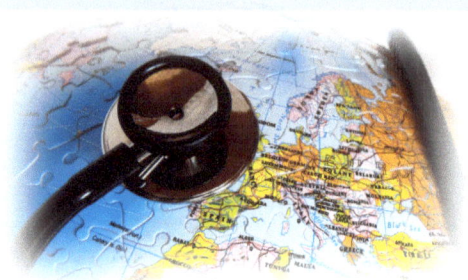

## ANCA

**Antineutrophil cytoplasmic antibodies** (ANCA) is associated with ILD:
(1) c-ANCA: GPA or Wegener granulomatosis
(2) p-ANCA EGPA or Churg–Strauss syndrome
(3) May be positive in anti-GBM antibody or Goodpasture disease

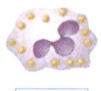
c-ANCA

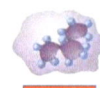
p-ANCA

# 19 Coal Worker's Pneumoconiosis

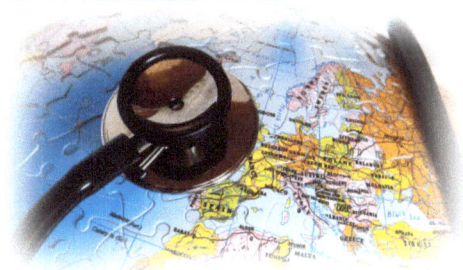

## Coal Worker's Pneumoconiosis

**Most patients with have no significant respiratory disability.**
Some patients may develop complicated pneumoconiosis, which is characterized by fibrosis. (Restrictive lung disease).
Caused by inhalation of coal dust, which contains carbon and silica.

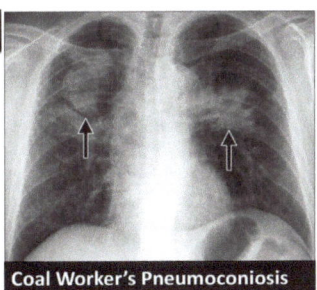

Coal Worker's Pneumoconiosis

# 20 Asbestosis

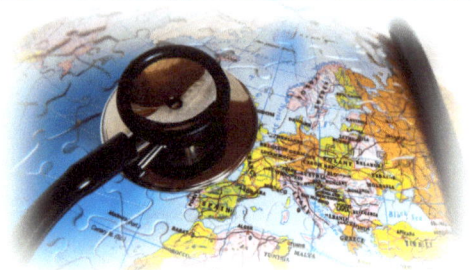

## Asbestosis

Characterized by diffuse interstitial fibrosis of the lung caused by inhalation of asbestos fibers. More prominent in the **lower lung lobes**. Develops gradually over many years >15 to 20 years after exposure. Diagnosis is made based on clinical findings (dyspnea) and history of exposure to asbestos.
CXR shows show **pleural plaques** (especially in lower lung regions).
No specific treatment is available.

**Increased risk of:**
**(1)** Bronchogenic carcinoma (smoking is synergistic)
**(2)** Malignant mesothelioma.

## Asbestosis

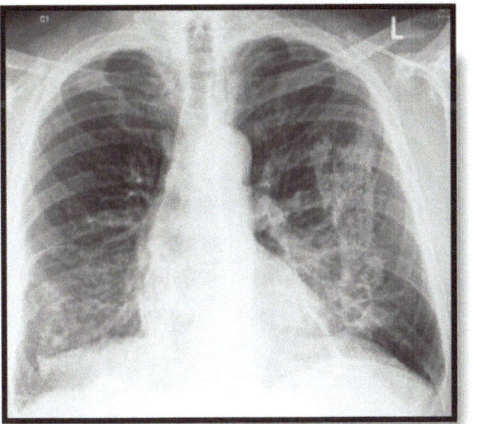

CXR in asbestosis showing **pleural plaques**

# 21 Silicosis

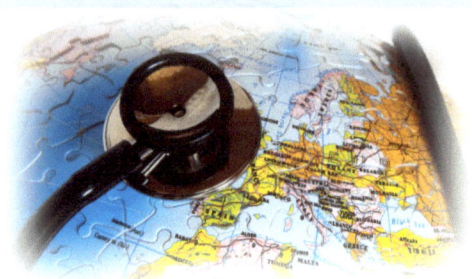

## Silicosis

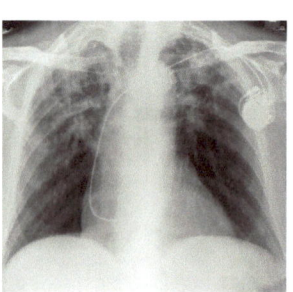

**Upper lobes** fibrosis- more common.
**Increased risk of TB**.
Sources include mining, stone cutting, and glass manufacturing.
Exertional dyspnea is the main symptom
Cough with sputum is also seen.
Restrictive pulmonary function abnormalities.
Treatment is removal from exposure to silica.

# 22 Berylliosis

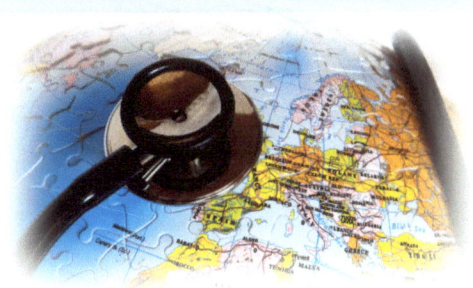

## Berylliosis

Very similar to sarcoidosis- granulomas, skin lesions. Hypercalcemia may be present. The beryllium lymphocyte proliferation test is a useful diagnostic blood test.
Treatment is glucocorticoid therapy for both acute and chronic berylliosis.

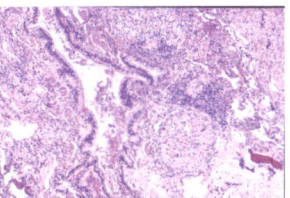

**C/P: Dry coughing, Dyspnea, Chest pain, Fatigue, Fever, Night sweats, Anorexia, Weight loss, Enlargement of lymph nodes.**

# 23 Hypersensitivity Pneumonitis

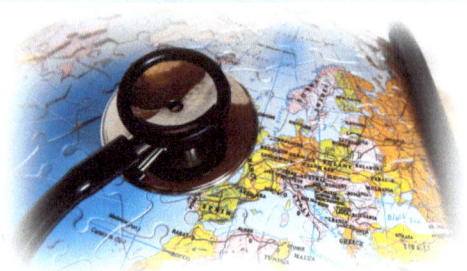

## Hypersensitivity Pneumonitis

Inhalation of an antigenic agent to the alveolar level induces an immune-mediated pneumonitis. Chronic exposure may lead to restrictive lung disease.
The presence of serum **IgG and IgA** against the inhaled antigen is a hallmark finding.
Acute form has flu-like features (fever, chills, cough, dyspnea).
CXR during the acute phase shows pulmonary infiltrates.

## Extrinsic Allergic Alveolitis

Treatment involves removal of the offending agent ± glucocorticoids.

## Hypersensitivity Pneumonitis

**Some causes of hypersensitivity pneumonitis:**
Farmer's lung (Moldy hay)
Bird-breeder's lung (Avian droppings)
Air-conditioner lung
Bagassosis (Moldy sugar cane)
Mushroom worker's lung (Compost)

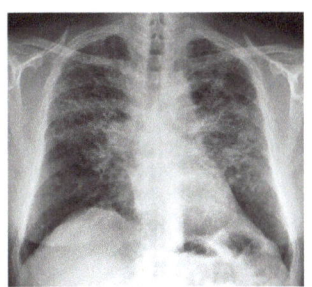

# 24 Eosinophilic Pneumonia

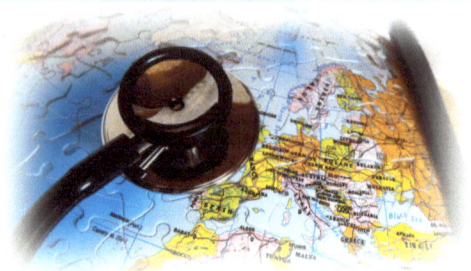

## Hypersensitivity Pneumonitis

**Some causes of hypersensitivity pneumonitis:**
Farmer's lung (Moldy hay)
Bird-breeder's lung (Avian droppings)
Air-conditioner lung
Bagassosis (Moldy sugar cane)
Mushroom worker's lung (Compost)

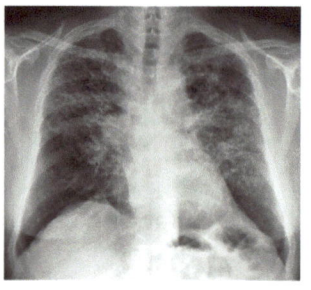

# 25 Goodpasture Disease

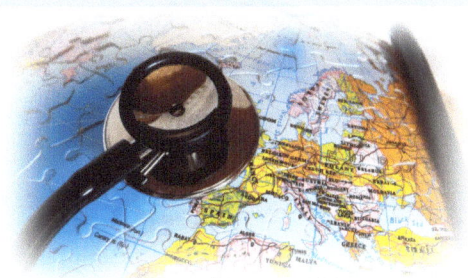

## Goodpasture Disease

Autoimmune disease caused by IgG antibodies directed against glomerular and alveolar basement membranes.
Usually presents with **hemoptysis and dyspnea**
Diagnosis made by tissue biopsy, serologic evidence of antiglomerular basement membrane antibodies.
Treatment include plasmapheresis, cyclophosphamide, and corticosteroids.

Anti-GBM Antibody or Goodpasture Disease: Hemoptysis *Plus* Hematuria

# 26 Pulmonary Alveolar Proteinosis

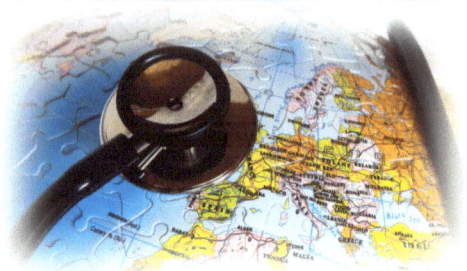

## Pulmonary Alveolar Proteinosis

Accumulation of surfactant-like protein and phospholipids in the alveoli. Usually presents with dry cough, dyspnea, hypoxia, and rales. CXR typically has a ground-glass appearance with bilateral alveolar infiltrates (a bat wing shape).
Lung biopsy is needed for definitive diagnosis.
**Treatment** is with lung lavage and granulocyte colony–stimulating factor.

Patients are at increased risk of infection, and corticosteroids should not be used.

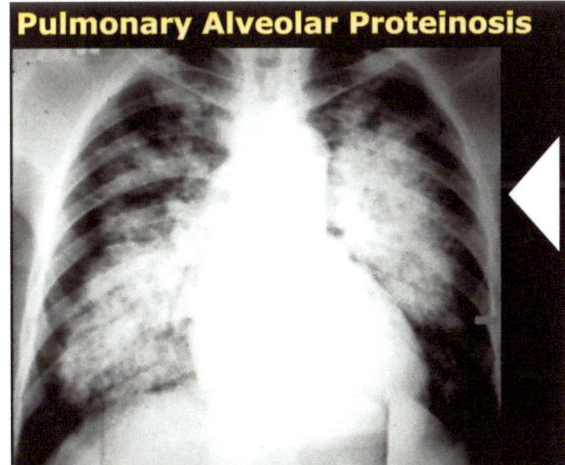 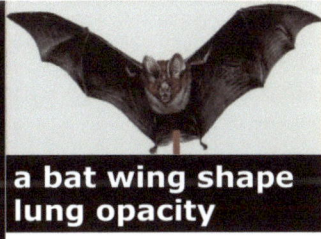

# 27 Idiopathic Pulmonary Fibro (IPF)

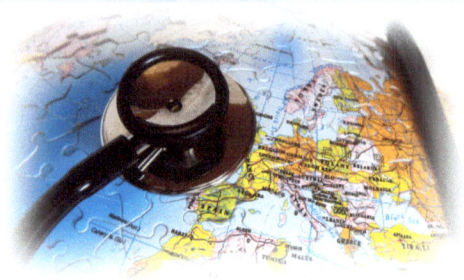

## Idiopathic Pulmonary Fibrosis

Etiology unknown.
More common in men and smokers.
Presents with gradual onset of progressive dyspnea and nonproductive cough.
Mean survival is only 3 to 7 years after first diagnosis.

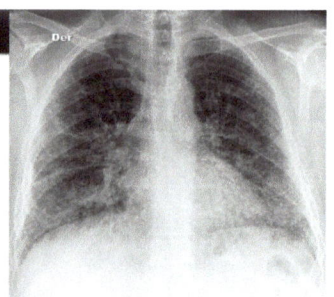

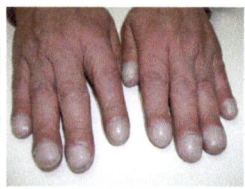

## Idiopathic Pulmonary Fibrosis
**Other causes of ILD must be excluded.**

**Chest X Ray:** ground-glass or a honeycombed appearance
**High-resolution CT of chest**
Definitive diagnosis requires open **lung biopsy** consistent with usual interstitial pneumonia.

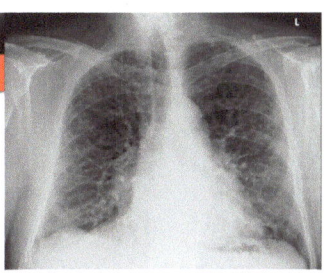

## Idiopathic Pulmonary Fibrosis

The **majority** of patients (>70%) do not improve with therapy and experience progressive and gradual respiratory failure.
Corticosteroids have been used historically but with little or no benefit and have significant side effects.
Lung transplantation is a treatment option.

**New anti-fibrotic agents:**
**Nintedanib** or **Pirfenidone** have been shown in trials to slow progression of mild and moderate disease.

# 28 Cryptogenic Organizing Pneumonitis

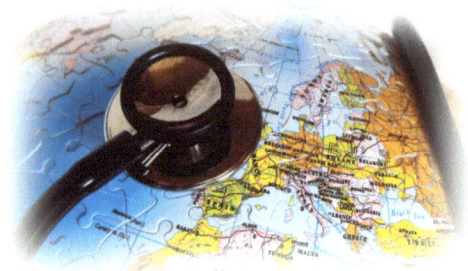

## Cryptogenic Organizing Pneumonitis

An inflammatory lung disease with similar clinical and radiographic features to infectious pneumonia. Associated with many entities (viral infections, medications, connective tissue disease).
Most cases are idiopathic.
Antibiotics have not been found to be effective.
**Corticosteroids** are used most commonly (>60% of patients recover).

Features include cough, dyspnea, and flu-like symptoms; bilateral patchy infiltrates on CXR.

# 29 Acute Respiratory Failure

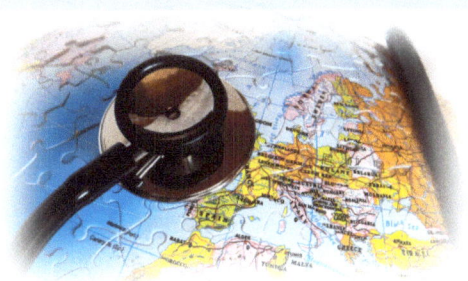

## Acute Respiratory Failure

**Definition:**
Hypoxia (PaO2 <60 mm Hg)
Hypercapnia (partial pressure of CO2 [PCO2] >50 mm Hg)

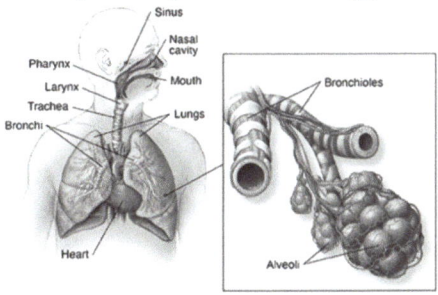

## Acute Respiratory Failure

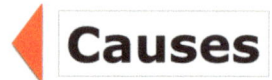 **Causes**

**CNS** (brain and spinal cord) depression or damage
**Neuromuscular disease**—myasthenia gravis, polio, Guillain–Barré syndrome.
**Upper airway**—obstruction e.g. stenoses, spasms, or paralysis
**Thorax and pleura**—mechanical restriction (kyphoscoliosis, flail chest, hemothorax)
**Cardiovascular system**—CHF, valvular diseases, PE, anemia
**Lower airways and alveoli**—asthma, COPD, pneumonia, acute respiratory distress syndrome (ARDS)

## Acute Respiratory Failure

To determine the underlying mechanism of hypoxemia **You need to know:**
PaCO2 level
A–a gradient
Response to supplemental oxygen

## Acute Respiratory Failure

**Hypoventilation:**
A–a gradient is normal

**V/Q mismatch or shunting:**
Both PaCO2 and A–a gradient are elevated

**Hypoxia due to a shunt is not responsive to supplemental oxygen.**

## Acute Respiratory Failure

A–a gradient is **Normal**

**Hypoventilation**

**Hypoventilation**—leads to **Hypoxemia + Hypercapnia**

**Note: Increased CO2 production** (e.g., sepsis, DKA, hyperthermia) results in **Hypercapnia.**

**Causes of hypoventilation:**
Central nervous system depression
Neurological disease
Disorders of the respiratory muscles
Severe Obesity

## Acute Respiratory Failure

**V/Q mismatch**
**Caused by** a defect in either Alveolar ventilation (pulmonary edema- COPD- Lung diseases) OR/ Perfusion (Pulmonary embolism)
**Typically** leads to **Hypoxia without Hypercapnia**

**V/Q mismatch Responds to supplemental oxygen**

V/Q mismatch is the most common mechanism of hypoxemia (especially in chronic lung disorders)

## Acute Respiratory Failure

**Shunting**
**Causes of shunts:**
Atelectasis or fluid buildup in alveoli (pneumonia or pulmonary edema), Direct right-to-left intracardiac blood flow in congenital heart diseases.

**Shunting Does Not respond to supplemental oxygen.**

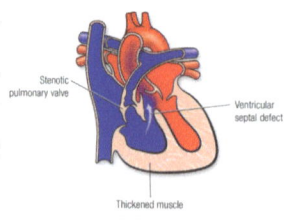
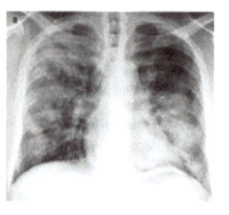

## Acute Respiratory Failure

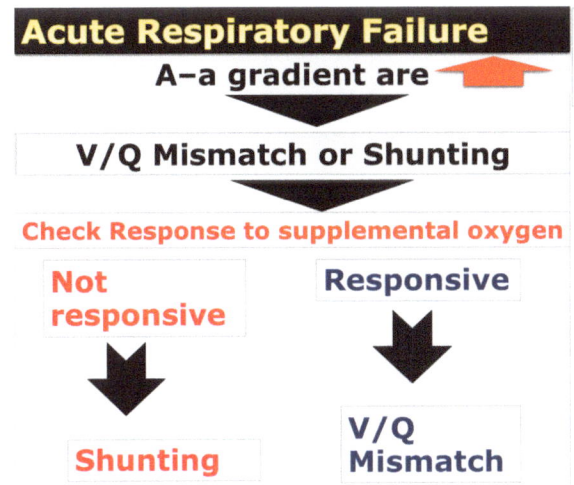

A–a gradient is Normal in hypoventilation.

## Acute Respiratory Failure

**Hypoxemic respiratory failure: Use the lowest concentration of oxygen** that provides sufficient oxygenation to avoid oxygen toxicity, which is due to free-radical production.

# 30. Acute Respiratory Distress Syndrome (ARDS)

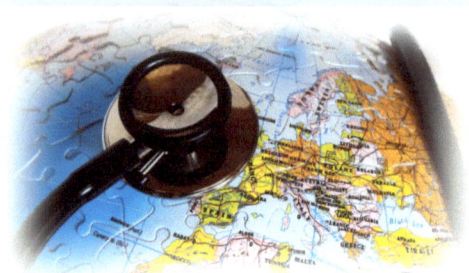

## ARDS

### Acute Respiratory Distress Syndrome

ARDS is a diffuse inflammatory process involving both lungs. Neutrophil activation in the systemic or pulmonary circulations is the main mechanism of the condition.

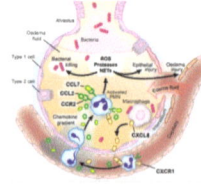

> ARDS is not a primary disease but a disorder that occurs due to other conditions that cause widespread inflammatory process.

## ARDS

**Caused of ARDS include:**
Sepsis
Aspiration of gastric contents
Severe trauma
Acute pancreatitis,
Multiple or massive transfusions
Drug overdose
Toxic inhalation
Intracranial HTN

Patients with Sepsis have the highest risk of developing ARDS (e.g., Pneumonia, Renal infections, Wound infections)

## ARDS

Massive intrapulmonary **shunting** of blood is a key pathophysiologic event in ARDS. It causes severe hypoxemia with **No improvement on 100% oxygen**.
Shunting is secondary to widespread atelectasis, collapse of alveoli, and surfactant dysfunction.

1) An increase in alveolar–capillary permeability causes ARDS
2) Congestive hydrostatic forces cause cardiogenic pulmonary edema.

## ARDS

**Diagnosis:**
**(1)** Hypoxemia that is refractory to oxygen therapy: Ratio of PaO2/FiO2 200 to 300 is mild, 100 to 200 is moderate, and <100 is severe
**(2)** Bilateral diffuse pulmonary infiltrates on CXR
**(3)** No evidence of CHF clinically or PCWP ≤18 mm Hg
**(4)** Respiratory symptoms that develop within 1 week of known insult

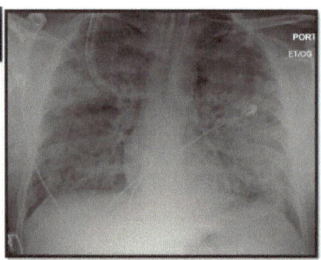

## ARDS

**Treatment:**
1) Oxygenation—try to keep O2 saturation >90%.
2) Mechanical ventilation
3) Volume overload should be avoided.
4) Do not forget to address the patient's nutritional needs (Tube feedings are preferred)
5) Treat the cause!

**Note:** Patients with sepsis have high fluid requirements

# 31 Mechanical Ventilation

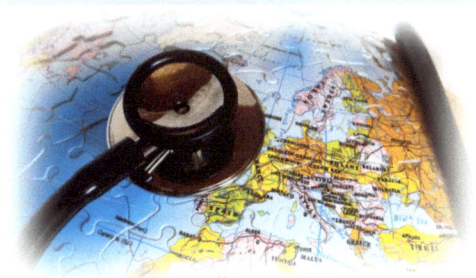

## Mechanical Ventilation

**Always** confirm correct ET placement by listening for bilateral breath sounds and checking a post-intubation CXR.

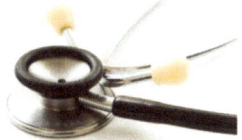

When a patient is ventilator dependent for 2 or more weeks, a **tracheostomy** is usually performed to prevent tracheomalacia.

# 32 Pulmonary Hypertension

## Pulmonary Hypertension

**Pulmonary Hypertension** (PH) Is defined as a mean pulmonary arterial pressure greater than 25 mm Hg at rest

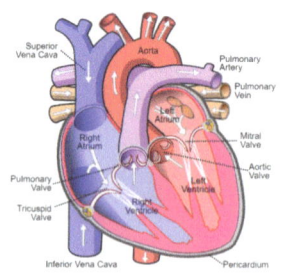

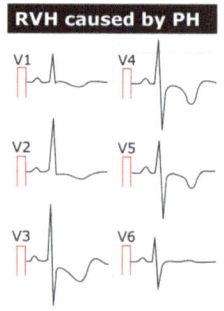

RVH caused by PH

## Pulmonary Hypertension

**Group 1:** Idiopathic Pulmonary arterial hypertension (PAH)
**Group 2:** Left heart disease (CHF-Mitral stenosis)
**Group 3:** Lung disease and/or chronic hypoxemia (COPD)
**Group 4:** Chronic thromboembolic disease (Recurrent PE)
**Group 5:** Miscellaneous Pulmonary vascular compression (e.g., tumors - lymphadenopathy – sarcoidosis)

## Pulmonary Hypertension

**Symptoms**
Dyspnea on exertion
Fatigue
Chest pain—exertional
Syncope—exertional (with severe disease)

**Signs**
Loud pulmonic component of the second heart sound (P2)

When **RVF** occurs, the corresponding signs and symptoms appear (JVD, hepatomegaly, ascites, peripheral edema).

## Pulmonary Hypertension

**ECG:** RVH
**CXR:** Dilated PA
**Echo**
**Right heart catheterization:** required for confirmatory diagnosis of pulmonary HTN. Reveals increased mean pulmonary artery pressure >25 mm Hg

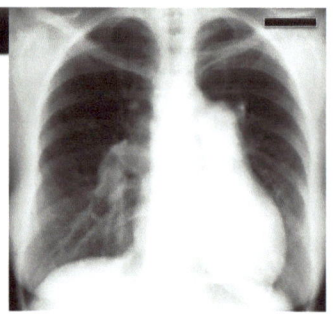

## Pulmonary Hypertension

If the pulmonary HTN is **Secondary** to another disease process (e.g., Recurrent PE) the underlying disease should be treated. Vasoactive agents are typically used in **Primary** PH (Idiopathic Pulmonary arterial hypertension), since some trials have been conducted in these patients.

**Many patients may need:**
Home oxygen
Diuretics
Inotropes (e.g., digoxin).

## Pulmonary Hypertension

**Note:** Vasoactive agents may lower pulmonary vascular resistance in some patients. Available options include inhaled nitric oxide, phosphodiesterase inhibitors (e.g., sildenafil), oral CCBs, prostacyclins (e.g., epoprostenol), and endothelin receptor antagonists (e.g., bosentan).

# 33 Cor Pulmonale

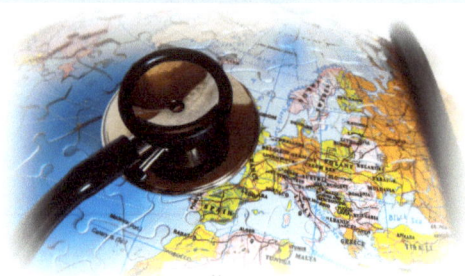

## Cor Pulmonale

**Definition: Right ventricular hypertrophy OR RV failure secondary to lung disease.**

### Clinical Picture:
Decrease in exercise tolerance
Cyanosis and digital clubbing
Signs of right ventricular failure: hepatomegaly, edema, JVD
Parasternal lift

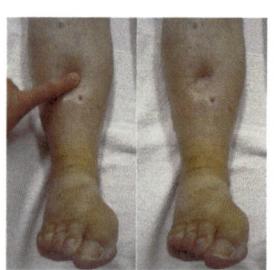

## Cor Pulmonale
**Treatment**
1) Treat the underlying pulmonary disorder.
2) Use diuretic therapy cautiously because patients may be preload dependent.
3) Apply continuous long-term oxygen therapy if the patient is hypoxic.
4) Administer digoxin **only** if there is coexistent LV failure.

# 34 Pulmonary Embolism (PE)

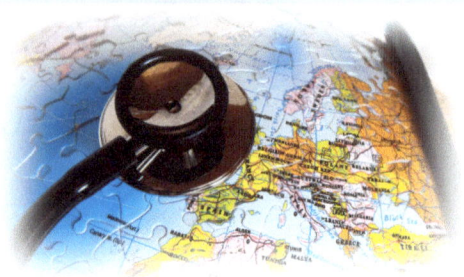

## Pulmonary Embolism

Pulmonary embolism occurs when a thrombus in another region of the body embolizes to the pulmonary vascular tree.

Most pulmonary emboli arise from thromboses in the deep veins of lower extremities above the knee (iliofemoral DVT).

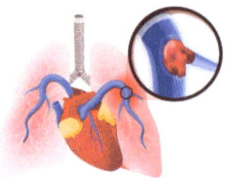

Most deaths in PE are due to recurrent PE within the first few hours of the initial embolism.

**Treatment with anticoagulants decreases the mortality by 95%.**

## Pulmonary Embolism

**Risk Factors for DVT/PE**
Age >60 years
Malignancy
Prior history of DVT, PE
Hereditary hypercoagulable states (factor V Leiden, protein C and S deficiency, antithrombin III deficiency)
Prolonged immobilization or bed rest, long-distance travel
Cardiac disease, especially CHF
Obesity
Nephrotic syndrome
Major surgery, especially pelvic surgery (orthopedic procedures)
Major trauma
Pregnancy, estrogen use (oral contraceptives)

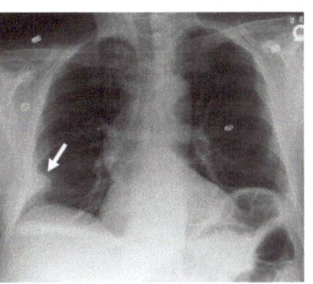

## Pulmonary Embolism

1) When PE is undiagnosed, mortality rate approaches 30%.
2) As many as 50% of cases are undiagnosed.
3) Treatment with **anticoagulants** decreases the mortality by 95%.

Most deaths are due to recurrent PE within the first few hours of the initial PE.

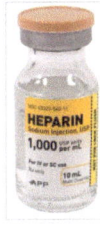
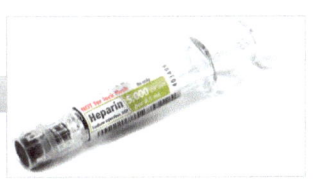

## Pulmonary Embolism

**Symptoms of Pulmonary Embolism:**
(According to PIOPED study)
1. **Dyspnea** (73%)
2. **Pleuritic chest pain** (66%)
3. Cough (37%)
4. Hemoptysis (13%)

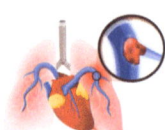

**Syncope + Shock is seen in large PE**

Only 1/3 of patients with PE will have signs and symptoms of a DVT

## Pulmonary Embolism

**Signs of Pulmonary Embolism:**
(According to PIOPED study)
Tachypnea (70%)
Rales (51%)
Tachycardia (30%)
S4 (24%)
Increased P2 (23%)
Other signs: low-grade fever, decreased breath sounds, dullness on percussion

**Syncope + Shock is seen in large PE**

If the patient has symptoms of PE and a DVT is found, You can make the diagnosis of PE **without** further testing.

## Pulmonary Embolism

(1) ABG levels are **not diagnostic** for Pulmonary Embolism
(2) CXR—usually normal
**(3) Venous duplex ultrasound of the lower extremities.**
If there is a positive result, treat with IV anticoagulation (heparin); treatment of DVT is the same as for PE. This test is very helpful when positive, but of little value when negative (negative results occur in 50% of patients with proven PE).

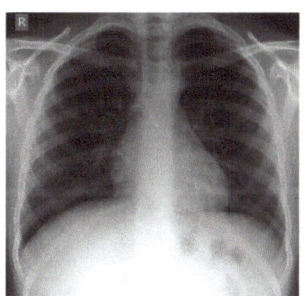

## Pulmonary Embolism

**V/Q (ventilation–perfusion lung) scan**
Traditionally, this was the most common test used when PE is suspected but has been replaced by **CT angiography** (CTA) as the initial study of choice in many medical centers. Plays an important role in diagnosis when there is a contraindication to CTA.

## Pulmonary Embolism

**1** A high-probability V/Q scan has a very high sensitivity for PE: **Treat with heparin.**

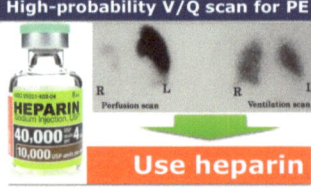

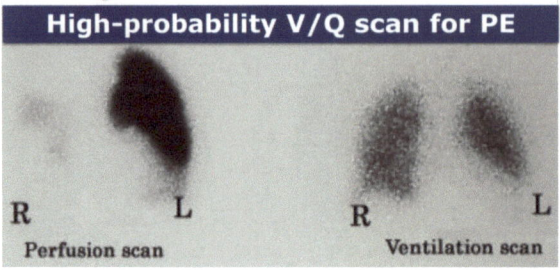

## Pulmonary Embolism

**2** If there is low probability of PE on V/Q lung scan, **clinical suspicion** determines the next step. **Check Duplex Results:**

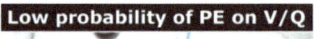

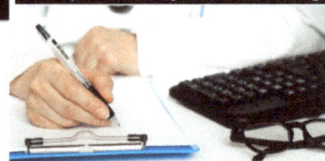

**Clinical suspicion Determines the Next Step!**

| If the **duplex** is **Positive** | If the duplex is **Negative** |
|---|---|
| 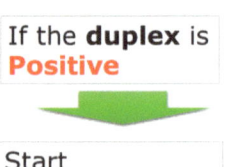 | 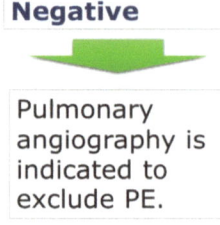 |
| Start anticoagulation. | Pulmonary angiography is indicated to exclude PE. |

## Pulmonary Embolism

**CTA (CT Angiography)**
Has good sensitivity (>90%) and specificity.
Can visualize very small clots (as small as 2 mm)
The **test of choice** in most medical centers.

If CTA is negative for PE, and clinical probability of PE is high, there is a **5% incidence of PE.**

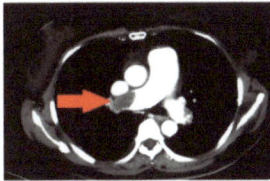

CTA (CT Angiography) is the test of choice for suspected Pulmonary Embolism PE

## Pulmonary Embolism

**CTA (CT Angiography)**
**Avoid** in patients with significant renal insufficiency because of the IV contrast that is required.

If CTA is negative for PE, and clinical probability of PE is high, there is a **5% incidence of PE**.

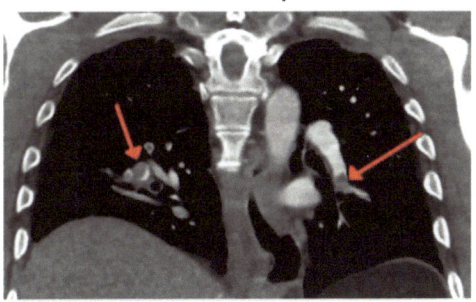

## Pulmonary Embolism

**Pulmonary angiography** is the most accurate tool in diagnosing PE But rarely used today as it carries a 0.5% mortality.

**Consider it in the following cases:**
(1) Noninvasive testing is equivocal Plus Risk of anticoagulation is high OR/
(2) If the patient is hemodynamically unstable, and embolectomy may be required.

**Pulmonary angiography Carries a 0.5% mortality**

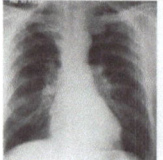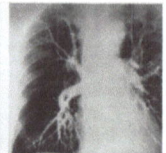

## Pulmonary Embolism

**D-dimer assay**
D-dimer is a specific fibrin degradation product.
It can be elevated in patients with PE and DVT.
D-dimer assay is a very **sensitive** test (90% to 98%) but NOT Specific.

**Specificity is low**—
D-dimer results may also be elevated in MI, CHF, pneumonia, and the postoperative state (or in any state of acute inflammation).

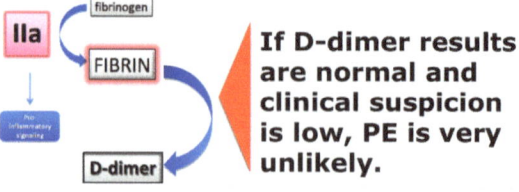

If D-dimer results are normal and clinical suspicion is low, PE is very unlikely.

## Pulmonary Embolism

**What does high sensitivity and low specificity D-dimer assay in Pulmonary Embolism mean?**

**If D-dimer is negative, you can rule out a clot.**

But if it is positive, it **does not prove** Pulmonary Embolism as many other conditions such as MI, CHF, and pneumonia can cause its elevation.

## Pulmonary Embolism

**Dichotomized Clinical Decision Rule for Suspected Acute Pulmonary Embolism (Modified Wells Criteria)**

| Factor | Points |
| --- | --- |
| Symptoms and signs of DVT | 3.0 |
| Alternative diagnosis less likely than PE | 3.0 |
| Heart rate >100 beats/min | 1.5 |
| Immobilization (>3 days) or surgery in previous 4 wks | 1.5 |
| Previous DVT or PE | 1.5 |
| Hemoptysis | 1.0 |
| Malignancy (current therapy, or in previous 6 months, or palliative) | 1.0 |

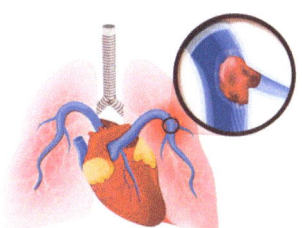

Adapted from Wells PS, Anderson DR, Rodger M, et al. Derivation of a simple clinical model to categorize patients probability of pulmonary embolism: increasing the models utility with the SimpliRED D-dimer. *Thromb Haemost* 2000;83(3):416–420.

**Score More than 4 : PE Likely**

## Pulmonary Embolism

**Acute anticoagulation therapy** with either unfractionated or low–molecular-weight heparin to prevent another PE.

Use Supplemental oxygen to correct hypoxemia

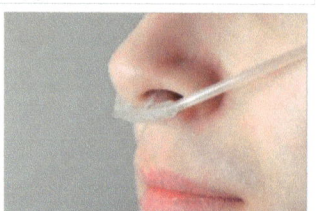

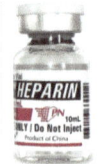

**Start immediately on basis of clinical suspicion. Do not wait for studies to confirm PE if clinical suspicion is high.**

For unfractionated heparin, give one bolus, followed by a continuous infusion for 5 to 10 days. The goal is an **aPTT of 1.5 to 2.5 times control.**

## Pulmonary Embolism

**Why PE and DVT are problematic for physicians:**
**(1)** Clinical findings are sometimes subtle in both.
**(2)** Noninvasive imaging tests do not always detect either condition.
**(3)** Anticoagulation carries significant risk.

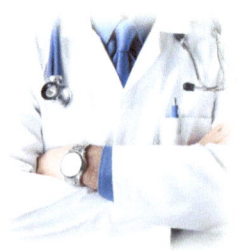

## Pulmonary Embolism

(1) **Heparin** acts by promoting the action of antithrombin III.
(2) Contraindications to heparin include active bleeding, uncontrolled HTN, recent stroke, and heparin-induced thrombocytopenia (HIT).
(2) Low–molecular-weight heparin has better bioavailability and lower complication rates than unfractionated heparin.

If anticoagulation is contraindicated in a patient with Pulmonary Embolism- **A Vena cava filter is indicated.**

## Pulmonary Embolism

**Oran anticoagulants:**
1) Long term anticoagulation for patients with PE is done by oral anticoagulation with warfarin or one of the novel oral anticoagulants (e.g., Rivaroxaban)
2) Continue for 3 to 6 months or more, depending on risk factors such as Malignancy and 3) Hypercoagulable state (may be considered for lifelong anticoagulation).

Target INR/PT with Warfarin treatment for PE is 2 to 3.

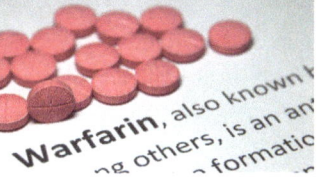

## Pulmonary Embolism

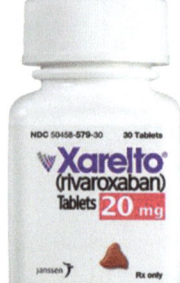

If you are using a novel oral anticoagulant (**Apixaban or Rivaroxaban**), premedication with heparin during initiation is not necessary as these medications are effective immediately.

**No need to premedicate with heparin when you use novel oral anticoagulants.**

### Rivaroxaban

## Pulmonary Embolism

**INR is a way of reporting the PT in a standardized fashion.**
Warfarin increases INR values. "Therapeutic" INR is usually between 2 and 3.

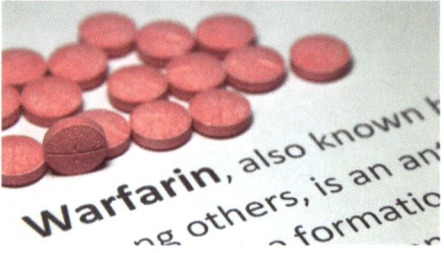

## Pulmonary Embolism

**Thrombolytic therapy for the treatment of Pulmonary Embolism (Streptokinase - tPA).** Speeds up the lysis of clots. Consider Thrombolytic therapy in the following situations:
**1)** Patients with massive PE who are hemodynamically unstable (e.g. Persistent hypotension).
**2)** Patients with evidence of right heart failure (thrombolysis can reverse this).

There is **no evidence** that thrombolysis improves mortality rates in patients with PE.

## Pulmonary Embolism

**Inferior vena cava interruption**
**Indications include:**
1) Contraindication to anticoagulation in a patient with documented DVT or PE.
2) A complication of current anticoagulation.
3) Failure of adequate anticoagulation as reflected by recurrent DVT or PE.
4) A patient with low pulmonary reserve who is at high risk for death from PE.

Use has become more common but reduction in mortality has not been conclusively demonstrated.

# 35 Pulmonary Aspiration

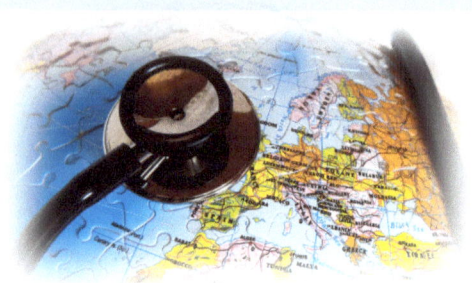

## Pulmonary Aspiration

The right lung is most often involved due to anatomy (right main bronchus follows a straighter path downward), particularly the lower segments of the right upper lobe and the upper segments of the right lower lobe.

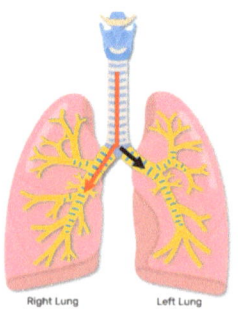

Aspiration pneumonia develops in 40% of patients who aspirate, usually 2 to 4 days after aspiration. Organisms are often mixed (aerobic–anaerobic).

## Pulmonary Aspiration

**Pulmonary aspiration syndromes can be due to different types of aspirates.**
1) Acidic gastric contents, which are especially damaging to the lungs.
2) Aspiration of oropharyngeal flora, which can lead to infection.
3) Foreign body/fluids (e.g., chemicals).

## Pulmonary Aspiration

Aspiration can lead to **lung abscess** if untreated. Poor oral hygiene predisposes to such infections. Foul-smelling sputum often indicates anaerobic infection.

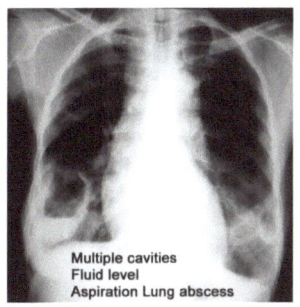

Multiple cavities
Fluid level
Aspiration Lung abscess

## Pulmonary Aspiration

**Treatment**
**(1)** If aspiration **pneumonia** is suspected, give antibiotics that have anaerobic activity (e.g., clindamycin).
**(2)** If **obstruction** is present, early bronchoscopy is indicated.
**(3)** Prevention is critical in patients at high risk for aspiration: Keep the head of the bed elevated.

**If aspiration occurred:**
ABCs (airway, breathing, and circulation), supplemental oxygen, and supportive measures.

# 36 Dyspnea

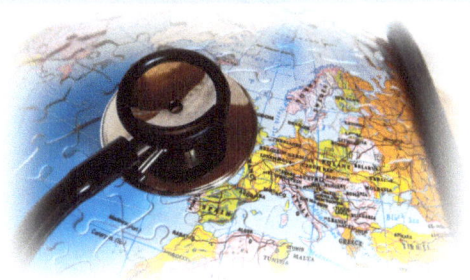

## Dyspnea

1) Patients with **chronic dyspnea** usually have either heart or lung disease or both.
2) The most common causes of **acute dyspnea** include CHF exacerbation, pneumonia, bronchospasm, Pulmonary Embolism, and anxiety.
3) If the patient has **a history of** smoking, cough, sputum, repeated infections, or occupational exposure, lung disease is likely to be the reason for chronic dyspnea.

## Dyspnea

Patients with chronic **COPD** can also experience paroxysmal nocturnal dyspnea due to accumulation of secretions.

Thus, paroxysmal nocturnal dyspnea (PND) is NOT specific to heart disease.

## Dyspnea

Depending on patient presentation, any of the following tests may be helpful in distinguishing between lung and heart diseases:
1) CXR
2) Sputum Gram stain and culture (if patient has sputum)
3) PFTs
4) ABGs
5) ECG, echocardiogram

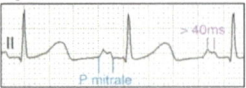

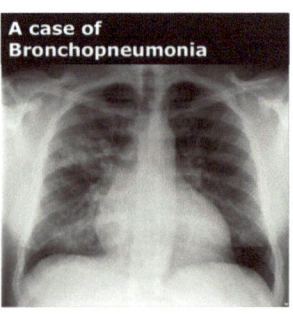

A case of Bronchopneumonia

# 37 Hemoptysis

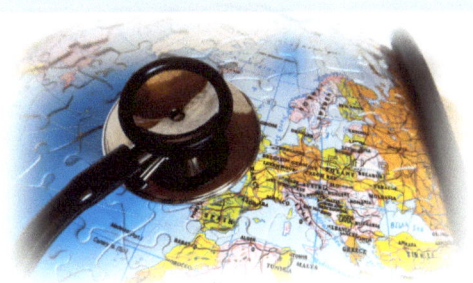

## Hemoptysis

**Most common causes of Hemoptysis include:**
Bronchitis (50% of cases)
Lung cancer (bronchogenic carcinoma)
TB
Bronchiectasis
Pneumonia
Many times the etiology remains idiopathic after thorough evaluation (up to 30% of cases)

**Other causes:**
Goodpasture syndrome)
Pulmonary Embolism with pulmonary infarction
Aspergilloma
Mitral stenosis
Hemophilia

## Hemoptysis

**History and physical Examination**
**(1)** Fever, night sweats, and weight loss suggest TB.
**(2)** Fevers and chills or a history of HIV suggests either pneumonia or TB.
**(3)** Look for risk factors for Pulmonary Embolism (PE).
**(4)** In the presence of acute renal failure or hematuria, Goodpasture syndrome should be considered.

Verify that hemoptysis has truly occurred.
**Note:** Superficial mouth lacerations, hematemesis, epistaxis, or may be confused with hemoptysis.

## Hemoptysis

**Chest X Ray**
May be a clear indicator of a pathogenic process or even diagnostic—For example, if fungus ball, irregular mass, granuloma, or opacity consistent with pulmonary infarction is present.

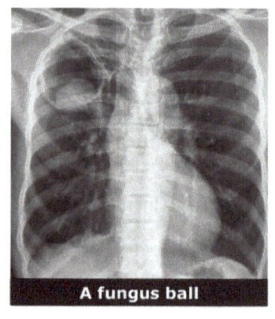
A fungus ball

A normal CXR does not exclude a serious cause of hemoptysis especially PE and even lung cancer.

## Hemoptysis
**Fiberoptic bronchoscopy**
Should be performed even if CXR is normal and if there is a significant clinical suspicion for lung carcinoma.

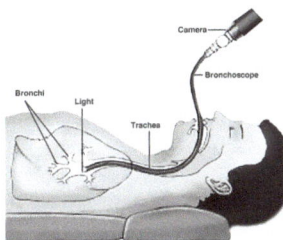

# 38. Pneumonia

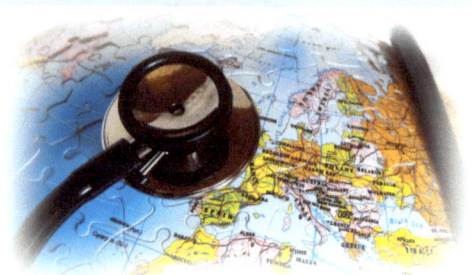

## Pneumonia

**Community Acquired Pneumonia** (CAP) presents with a sudden chill followed by fever, pleuritic pain, and productive cough.

**Most common** bacterial pathogen is **Streptococcus pneumoniae**

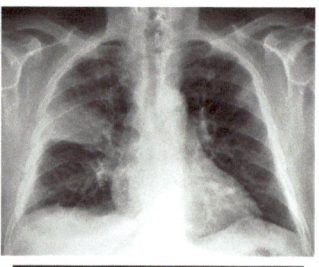
Streptococcus pneumoniae

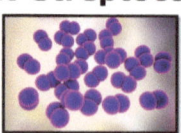

**Most cases** of CAP result from aspiration of oropharyngeal secretions.

## Pneumonia
### Prevention of CAP
**Influenza vaccine**—give yearly to people at increased risk for complications and to healthcare workers

**Pneumococcal vaccine**—for patients >65 years and for younger people at high risk (heart disease, sickle cell disease, pulmonary disease, diabetes, alcoholic cirrhosis, asplenia)

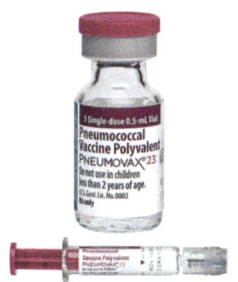

## Pneumonia
**Community Acquired Pneumonia** (CAP) presents with a sudden chill followed by fever, pleuritic pain, and productive cough.
**Most common** bacterial pathogen is **Streptococcus pneumoniae**

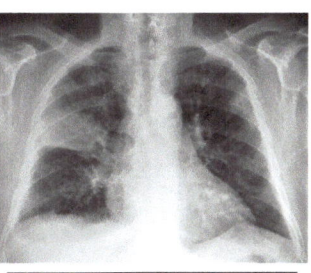

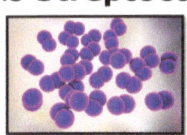

**Most cases** of CAP result from aspiration of oropharyngeal secretions.

## Pneumonia

**Nosocomial pneumonia
Occurs during hospitalization after first 72 hours**
Most common bacterial pathogens are **gram-negative rods** (Escherichia coli, Pseudomonas) and Staphylococcus aureus

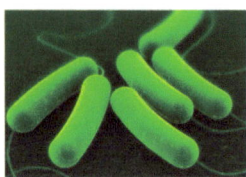

## Pneumonia

**S. pneumoniae accounts for up to 66% of all cases of bacteremic pneumonia**, followed by H. influenzae, influenza virus, and Legionella spp.

**Note:** Streptococcus pneumoniae bacteria cause pneumococcal disease, but are also commonly found in the respiratory track of healthy people

## Pneumonia

Studies have shown that if **vital signs** are entirely normal, the probability of pneumonia in outpatients is less than 1%.

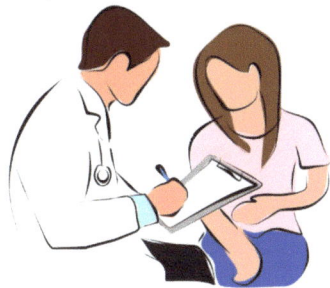

## Pneumonia

**Predisposing factors:**
❶ Loss of cough reflex : Coma- Anesthesia- Neuromuscular disease.
❷ Injury to the Mucociliary apparatus such as Cigarette smoking- Viral diseases- Immotile Cilia Syndrome (associated with Infertility)
❸ Inhibition of the phagocytic activity in the lung: Alcohol- D.M.- Immunosuppression
❹ Pulmonary congestion: LSHF
❺ Stasis of lung secretions: Cystic Fibrosis

> **Predisposing factors of pneumonia**

## Pneumonia

**Sputum studies (sputum acid-fast testing)**
(1) Definitive diagnosis is made by sputum culture—growth of M. tuberculosis
(2) Obtain three morning sputum specimens—culture takes 4 to 8 weeks
(3) PCR can detect specific mycobacterial DNA more rapidly

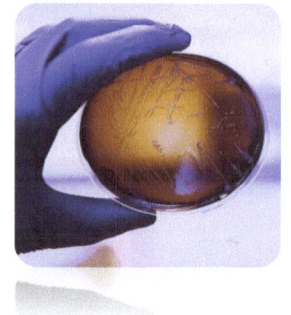

## Pneumonia

**Community Acquired Pneumonia CAP**

**Symptoms**
Acute onset of fever and shaking chills
Cough productive of thick, purulent sputum
Pleuritic chest pain (suggests the presence of pleural effusion)
Dyspnea

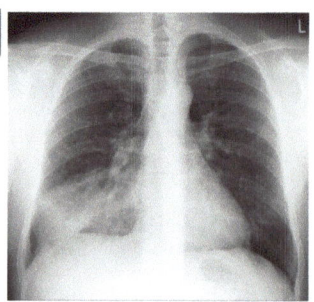

## Pneumonia

**Community Acquired Pneumonia CAP**

**Signs**
Tachycardia, tachypnea
Late inspiratory crackles, bronchial breath sounds, increased tactile and vocal fremitus, dullness on percussion
Pleural friction rub (associated with pleural effusion)

## Pneumonia

**Sputum Culture**
**CAP**
The value of routine sputum collection for Gram stain and culture is controversial.

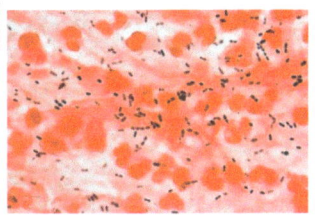

The **Infectious Disease Society of America** has recently advocated performing sputum Gram stain and culture in all patients hospitalized with CAP.

## Pneumonia

**CXR**
**(1)** Chest X Ray is considered sensitive for the diagnosis of pneumonia
**(2)** After treatment, changes evident on CXR usually lag behind the clinical response (up to 6 weeks).
**(3)** Changes include interstitial infiltrates, lobar consolidation, and/or cavitation.

**Important Note:**
If CXR findings are not suggestive of pneumonia, do not treat the patient with antibiotics.

## Pneumonia

**General Approach to Diagnosis of CAP**
The **first step** is to differentiate lower respiratory tract infection from the other causes of cough and from upper respiratory infection.
If nasal discharge, sore throat, or ear pain predominates, upper respiratory infection is likely.

## Pneumonia
### General Approach to Diagnosis of CAP
You must differentiate between pneumonia and acute bronchitis.

**Clinical features (cough, sputum, fever, dyspnea) are not reliable in differentiating between the two.**

### Note:
**CXR** is the only reasonable method of differentiating between pneumonia and acute bronchitis.

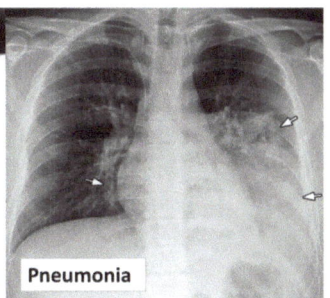
Pneumonia

## Pneumonia
Test for microbial diagnosis for outpatients is not required.
**Empiric treatment is often successful if CAP is suspected.**

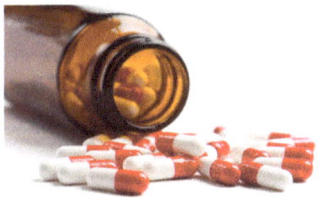

If patient is hypoxic or hypotensive, admit to hospital.

## Pneumonia

(1) In **alcoholics**, think of Klebsiella pneumoniae; in immigrants, think of TB.

(2) In **nursing homes**, consider a nosocomial pathogen (Pseudomonas).

**(3) Legionella pneumonia** is common in organ transplant recipients, Renal failure, Chronic lung disease, and Smokers and presents with GI symptoms and hyponatremia.

**Note:**
HIV-positive patients are at risk for P. carinii and M. tuberculosis but are still more likely to have a typical infectious agent.

## Pneumonia

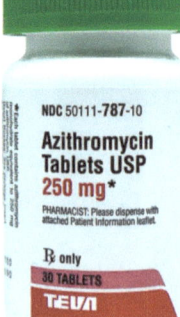

Treatment of **Uncomplicated CAP**

In patients without significant comorbidities, treat with:
**Azithromycin or Clarithromycin.**

◀ **Treatment of CAP**

## Pneumonia

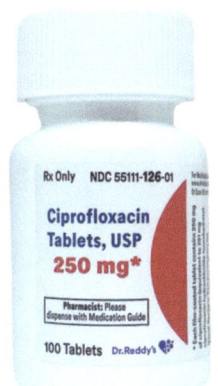

If the patient has **Comorbidities**: give a **Fluoroquinolone**.

Comorbidities of pneumonia: Hypertension, diabetes, obesity, asthma, immunosuppression, other CVDs, chronic obstructive pulmonary disease (COPD), and chronic kidney disease.

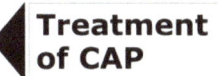

**Treatment of CAP**

## Pneumonia

**Outpatient treatment:**
In people younger than 60 years of age, Macrolides (azithromycin or clarithromycin) or doxycycline cover the most common organisms and are the first-line treatment. Fluoroquinolones are alternative agents.

**Penicillins or cephalosporins Do NOT cover the atypical organisms in this age group.**

In patients younger than 60 Ys old are the most common organisms are S. pneumoniae, Mycoplasma, Chlamydia, and Legionella.

## Pneumonia

**Outpatient treatment:**
In people younger than 60 years of age, Macrolides (azithromycin or clarithromycin) or doxycycline cover the most common organisms and are the first-line treatment. Fluoroquinolones are alternative agents.

**Penicillins or cephalosporins Do NOT cover the atypical organisms in this age group.**

In patients younger than 60 Ys old are the most common organisms are S. pneumoniae, Mycoplasma, Chlamydia, and Legionella.

## Pneumonia

**Outpatient treatment:**
Treatment is continued for **5 days**.

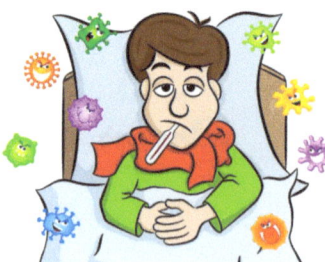

**Do not** stop treatment until patient has been afebrile for 48 hours.

## Pneumonia

For **hospitalized patients**, treatment is tailored toward gram-negative rods - a fluoroquinolone alone or a third-generation cephalosporin **PLUS** a macrolide.

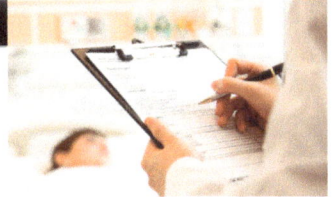

**For example:**
**Ceftriaxone + Azithromycin**

**Unlike CAP**, Macrolides are not used as single-agent therapy for hospital acquired pneumonia.

## Pneumonia

**Pleural effusion is common in patients with pneumonia**. Progression to empyema (infected, loculated pleural fluid) requires chest tube drainage.

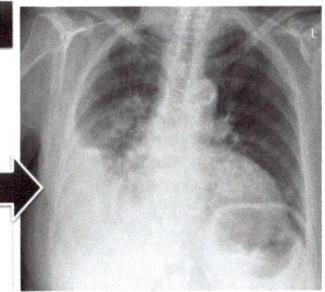

# 39 Pulmonary Tuberculosis

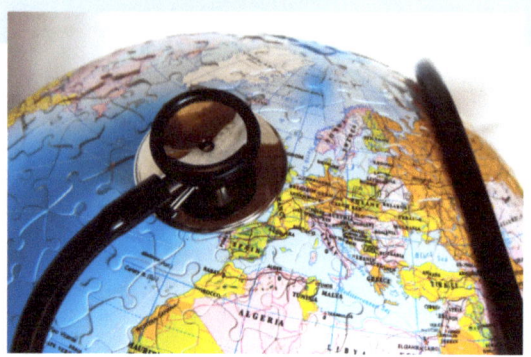

## Pulmonary Tuberculosis

Suspect it when there is Chronic chest complaints NOT responding to ordinary treatment

| Anorexia-Night Fever- Weakness- night sweats- Loss of Weight | Cough Expectoration Hemoptysis |
|---|---|

❶ Positive Tuberculin Test
❷ Apical pulmonary infiltrates
❸ Sputum smear examination with Z-N stain or
❹ Direct Florescence Studies
Positive Culture for the organism
❺ ↑↑↑ ESR

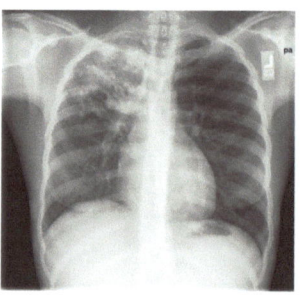

## Pulmonary Tuberculosis

Use combination chemotherapy of at least 4 Drugs of the following:

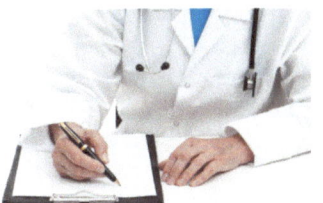

1. INH
2. Rifampicin
3. Pyrazinamide
4. Ethionamide
5. Streptomycin

## Pulmonary Tuberculosis

(1) Most Patients are effectively treated with 6 Months (or 9 Months) Chemotherapy.
(2) Monitor the treatment by Sputum Examination
(3) Corticosteroids are added to the treatment in cases of Tuberculous Meningitis (to decrease fibrosis)

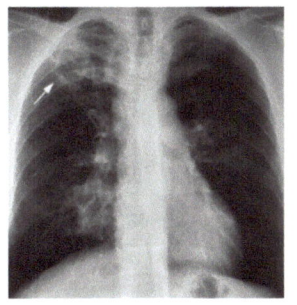

## Pulmonary Tuberculosis

**INH** should always be started with vitamin B6 (pyridoxine) to prevent Vitamin **B6 deficiency**.

**Symptoms of B6 deficiency:** stomatitis, glossitis, cheilosis, convulsions, hyperirritability, peripheral neuropathy, and sideroblastic anemia.

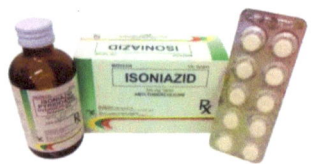

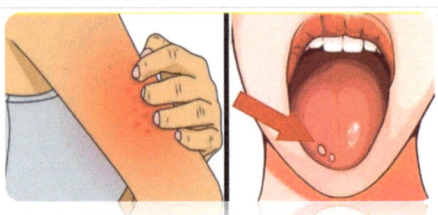

## Pulmonary Tuberculosis

TB is the most common cause of death due to infection **worldwide**.

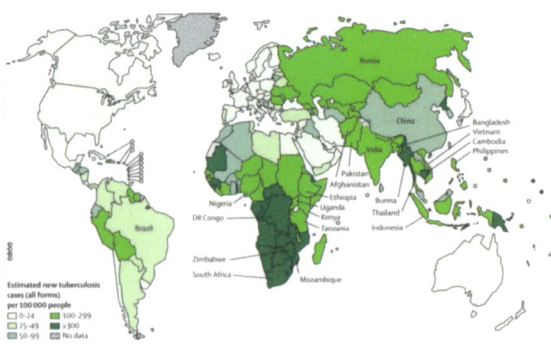

### Secondary T. B or Reactivation
Is seen when the host's immunity is weakened
HIV infection
Malignancy
Immunosuppressants
Substance abuse
Poor nutrition

## Pulmonary Tuberculosis

**Diagnosis of TB is challenging in HIV patients because:**
PPD skin test result is negative.
Patients have "atypical" CXR findings.
Sputum smears are more likely to be negative.
Granuloma formation may not be present in the late stages.

## Pulmonary Tuberculosis

**Clinical manifestations:**
Constitutional symptoms—fever, night sweats, weight loss, and malaise are common
Usually manifests in the most oxygenated portions of the lungs—the apical/posterior segments
T.B. is a differential diagnosis of almost all chest symptoms and signs.

You must have a **high index of suspicion**, depending on patient's risk factors and presentation

## Pulmonary Tuberculosis

(1) **INH** may lead to Pyridoxine deficiency which causes peripheral Neuropathy- Regular test for **Peripheral Neuropathy**!
Add Pyridoxine (Vitamin B6) to the treatment if INH is used.
(2) **Ethambutol** may cause **Optic Neuritis** (Test for Red & Green Vision)
(3) **Rifampicin & Pyrazinamide** may cause **hepatotoxicity** (Test for Liver Functions)

**Streptomycin** may damage the $8^{th}$ **Cranial Nerve** (Test for Vestibular functions)

## Pulmonary Tuberculosis

What does the presence of positive tuberculin test mean?

**Tuberculin Test**

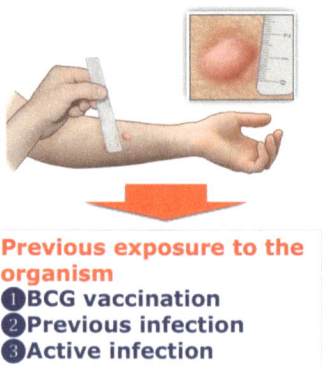

Previous exposure to the organism
① BCG vaccination
② Previous infection
③ Active infection

## Pulmonary Tuberculosis — Tuberculin Test

In people **without** any risk of tuberculosis

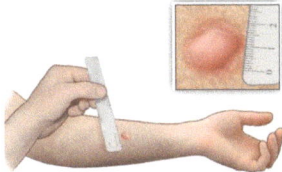

What is the diameter of the nodule in Tuberculin Test that suggests the presence of tuberculosis?

≥ **15 mm**

## Pulmonary Tuberculosis — Tuberculin Test

In any of these situations:

1. Newly emigrants
2. I.V. drug users
3. Chronic illness such as Diabetes Mellitus
4. Silicosis

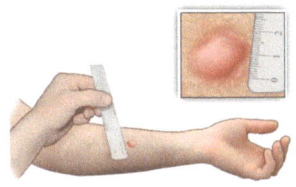

What is the diameter of the nodule in Tuberculin Test that suggests the presence of tuberculosis?

≥ **10 mm**

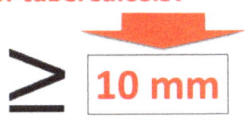

## Pulmonary Tuberculosis

### In any of these situations:

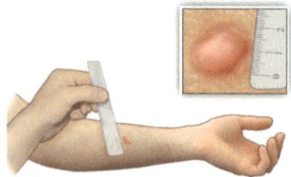

1. HIV positive,
2. Immunosuppressed
3. Recent exposure to patients with active tuberculosis

## Tuberculin Test

**What is the diameter of the nodule in Tuberculin Test that suggests the presence of tuberculosis?**

≥ 5 mm

# 40 Sleep Apnea Syndrome

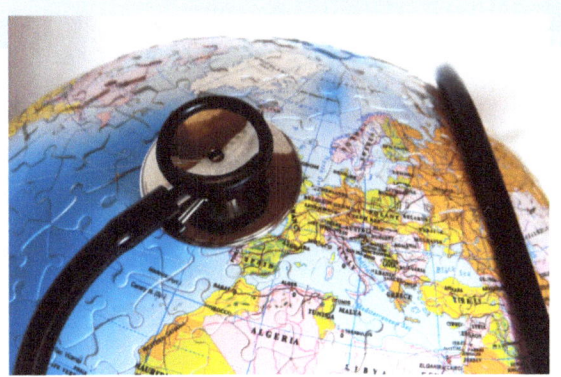

## Sleep Apnea Syndrome
Recurrent attacks of apnea during sleep that causes medical and health complications

**Manifestations:**
Snoring by night
Morning headache
Day time sleepiness
Impotence

**Ear Oximeter to detect the attacks of night hypoxemia**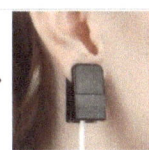

**If more severe it may lead to:**
1- Secondary polycythemia
2- Hypertension
3- Pulmonary Hypertension
4- Arrhythmias

## Sleep Apnea Syndrome

**Causes:**
1. Inhibition of the CNS
Alcohol
Sedatives
2. Narrowing of the pharyngeal lumen
Obesity
Acromegaly
Myxedema
3. Increased resistance to air flow proximal to pharynx
Allergic Rhinitis
Deviated Septum
Large tonsils or adenoids

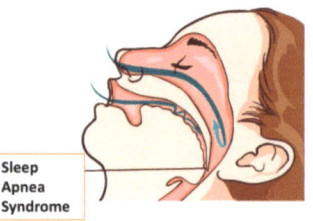

Sleep Apnea Syndrome

## Sleep Apnea Syndrome

1. Avoid Alcohol
2. Weight loss
3. Nasal CPAP to overcome proximal obstruction
4. Surgery in severe cases (Tracheostomy)

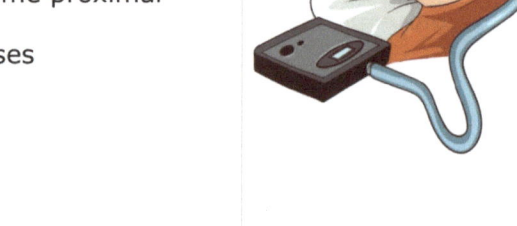

**In cases of COPD - If Polycythemia is much more than expected for a given degree of hypoxemia You must suspect associated Sleep apnea.**

# 41 Lung Abscess

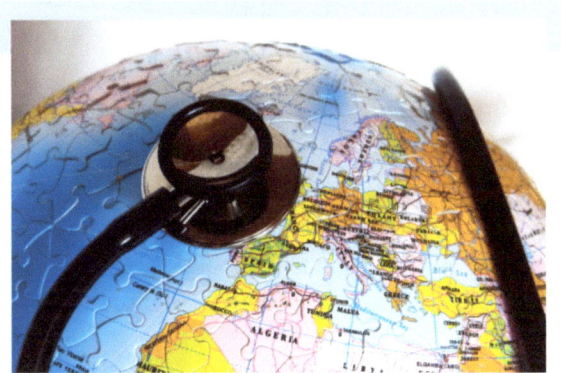

## Lung Abscess

The typical case is aspiration of a large volume of oropharyngeal contents or food causing pneumonia and necrosis.

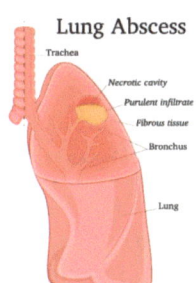

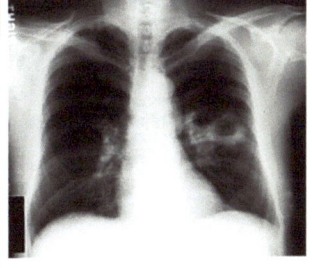

## Lung Abscess

The main risk factor is predisposition to aspiration.
This may be seen in patients with impaired consciousness (alcoholism, seizures), dysphagia, neurologic conditions (CVA), or mechanical disruption of normal defense mechanisms (nasogastric or endotracheal tube).

Poor dental hygiene increases the content of oral anaerobes.

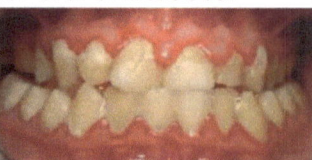

## Lung Abscess

**Symptoms of lung abscess:**
Cough—Foul-smelling sputum is consistent with anaerobic infection.
Expectoration of yellowish feted dependent discharge.
It is sometimes blood tinged.
Shortness of breath.
Fever, chills.
Constitutional symptoms: fatigue, malaise, weight loss.

## Lung Abscess

**CXR**
This reveals thick-walled cavitation with air–fluid levels.
**CT scan** may be necessary to differentiate between abscess and empyema.
**Note:** Sputum Gram stain and culture has low sensitivity and specificity.

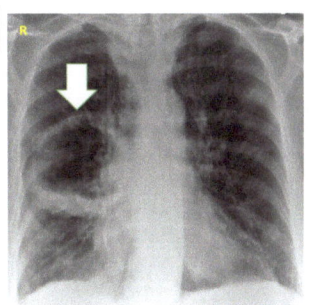

## Lung Abscess

**Treatment of lung abscess [1]**
**Antimicrobial therapy.**
Antibiotic regimens include coverage for the following:
Gram-positive cocci—
ampicillin/sulbactam or amoxicillin/clavulanic acid, ampicillin/sulbactam

**Note:** Use vancomycin for S. aureus

Hospitalization is often required if lung abscess is found.

**Postural drainage should be performed**

## Lung Abscess

**Treatment of lung abscess [2]**
**Anaerobes**—use Clindamycin or Metronidazole.
If **gram-negative organisms** are suspected, *add* a Fluoroquinolone or Ceftazidime.

Continue antibiotics **until** the cavity is gone or until CXR findings have improved considerably—this may take several months.

# 42 Bronchiectasis

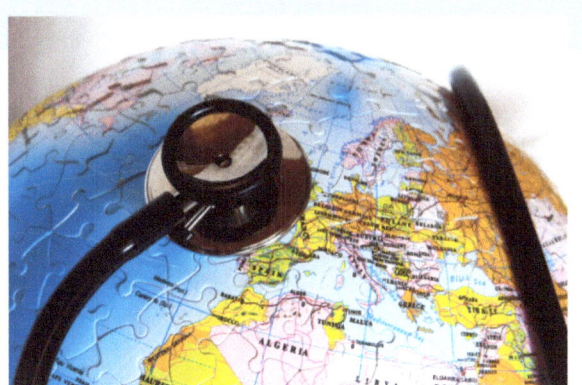

## Bronchiectasis

**Clinical features:**
Chronic persistent dilatation of the bronchi. **It can be associated with:**
1) Chronic cough with large amounts of mucopurulent, foul-smelling sputum
2) Dyspnea
3) Hemoptysis may occur due to rupture of blood vessels near bronchial wall surfaces
4) Recurrent pneumonia

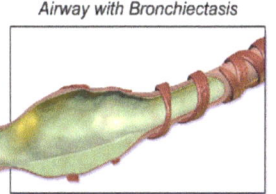
*Airway with Bronchiectasis*

## Bronchiectasis

High-resolution CT scan is the diagnostic study of choice.

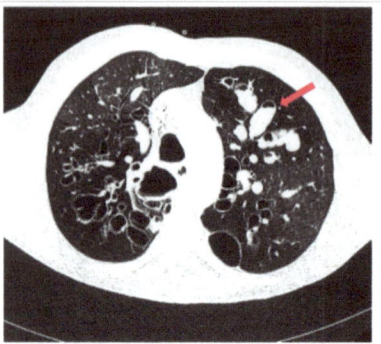

**Treatment:**
**Antibiotics for acute exacerbations + Bronchial hygiene**

## Bronchiectasis

CXR is abnormal in most cases, but findings are nonspecific.

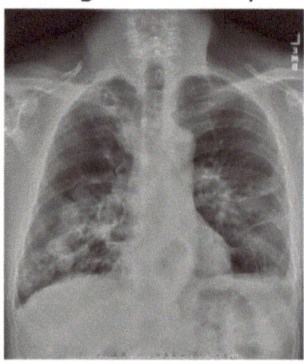

## Bronchiectasis

**Treatment:**
**Antibiotics for acute exacerbations— PLUS**
**Bronchial hygiene**
Hydration
Chest physiotherapy (postural drainage, chest percussion) to help remove the mucus
Inhaled bronchodilators

**Long-term antibiotics should be offered for adults with bronchiectasis who have three or more exacerbations per yr.**

Superimposed infections are signaled by change in quality/quantity of sputum, fever, or chest pain.

## Bronchiectasis

**Treatment:**
**Antibiotics for acute exacerbations— PLUS**
**Bronchial hygiene**

In patients with inadequate or inconclusive laboratory results, empiric therapy with amoxicillin/clavulanate, TMP-SMX, Doxycycline, a fluoroquinolone, or cefuroxime for 14 to 21 days is recommended

Pneumococcal vaccination and annual influenza vaccination is recommended for patients with chronic bronchiectasis.

www.ingramcontent.com/pod-product-compliance
Lightning Source LLC
Chambersburg PA
CBHW040217220526
45473CB00001B/14